EAT DAIRY FREE
SOUS VIDE
COOKBOOK

 Simple, Satisfying Recipes. The Ultimate Cookbook for Lactose Intolerance, Milk Allergies, and Casein-Free Living.

Sophia Marchesi

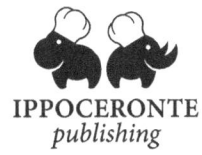

IPPOCERONTE
publishing

Copyright © 2021 by Sophia Marchesi
All rights reserved

This document is geared towards providing exact and reliable information with regards to the topic and issue covered. The publication is sold with the idea that the publisher is not required to render accounting, officially permitted, or otherwise, qualified services. If advice is necessary, legal or professional, a practiced individual in the profession should be ordered.

From a Declaration of Principles which was accepted and approved equally by a Committee of the American Bar Association and a Committee of Publishers and Associations.

In no way is it legal to reproduce, duplicate, or transmit any part of this document in either electronic means or in printed format. Recording of this publication is strictly prohibited and any storage of this document is not allowed unless with the written permission from the publisher. All rights reserved.

The information provided herein is stated to be truthful and consistent, in that liability, in terms of inattention or otherwise, by any usage or abuse of any policies, processes, or directions contained within is the solitary and utter responsibility of the recipient reader. Under no circumstances will any legal responsibility or blame be held against the publisher for any reparation, damages, or monetary loss due to the information herein, either directly or indirectly.

Respective authors own all copyrights not held by the publisher.

The information herein is offered for informational purposes solely and is universal as so. The presentation of the information is without a contract or any type of guarantee assurance.

The trademarks that are used are without any consent, and the publication of the trademark is without permission or backing by the trademark owner. All trademarks and brands within this book are for clarifying purposes only and are owned by the owners themselves, not affiliated with this document.

CONTENTS

INTRODUCTION 7
RECIPES 11
1. Crispy Egg Yolks 12
2. Eggs and Oregano 14
3. Cocktail Meatballs 16
4. White Bean and Artichoke Dip 18
5. Salty Custard 20
6. Spring Onion Soup 22
7. Spring Minestrone Soup 24
8. Mushroom Orzo Green Soup 26
9. Potato and Curry Soup 28
10. Bourbon Chicken 30
11. Lemon Herb Turkey Breast 32
12. Arrowroot Country-Style Ribs 34
13. Beef Tri-Tip with BBQ Sauce 36
14. Herb Rub Pork Chops 38
15. Chopped Duck with Honey 40
16. BBQ Pork Ribs 42
17. Simple Sliced Pork Belly 44
18. Rosemary Garlic Lamb Chops 46
19. Bacon 48
20. Tempting Teriyaki Chicken 50
21. Spiced Lamb Kebabs 52
22. Simple Rack of Lamb 54
23. Blackened Brussels Sprouts with Garlic and Bacon 56
24. Huevos Rancheros 58
25. Cherry Tomatoes with Eggs 60
26. Shrimp and mushrooms 62

27. Sweet Paprika with Zucchini Prosciutto 64
28. Spring Vegetable Risotto.. 66
29. Garlicky Brussels Sprouts.. 68
30. Green Beans Almondine 69
31. Winter Vegetables 70
32. Garlicky Ratatouille.. 72
33. Garlic Mushrooms with Truffle Oil 74
34. Rosemary Potatoes... 76
35. Warm Assorted Broccoli Salad 78
36. Tangy Tender Mushrooms 80
37. Colorful Bell Pepper Mix 82
38. King Prawns with Ginger and Caramelized Onion 84
39. Caramel Shrimp Chili... 86
40. Cod... 88
41. Walnut Coated Halibut... 90
42. Salmon Fillets 92
43. East Asian Marinated Catfish... 94
44. Simple Honey Glazed Carrots 96
45. Spicy Pickled Vegetable Medley 98
46. Strawberry Jam.. 100
47. Strawberries with Balsamic Vinegar.............................. 102
48. Allspice Poached Pear 104
49. Raspberry Compote 106
50. Cinnamon Apples 107

TEMPERATURE CHARTS 108
COOKING CONVERSION 114
RECIPE INDEX 118

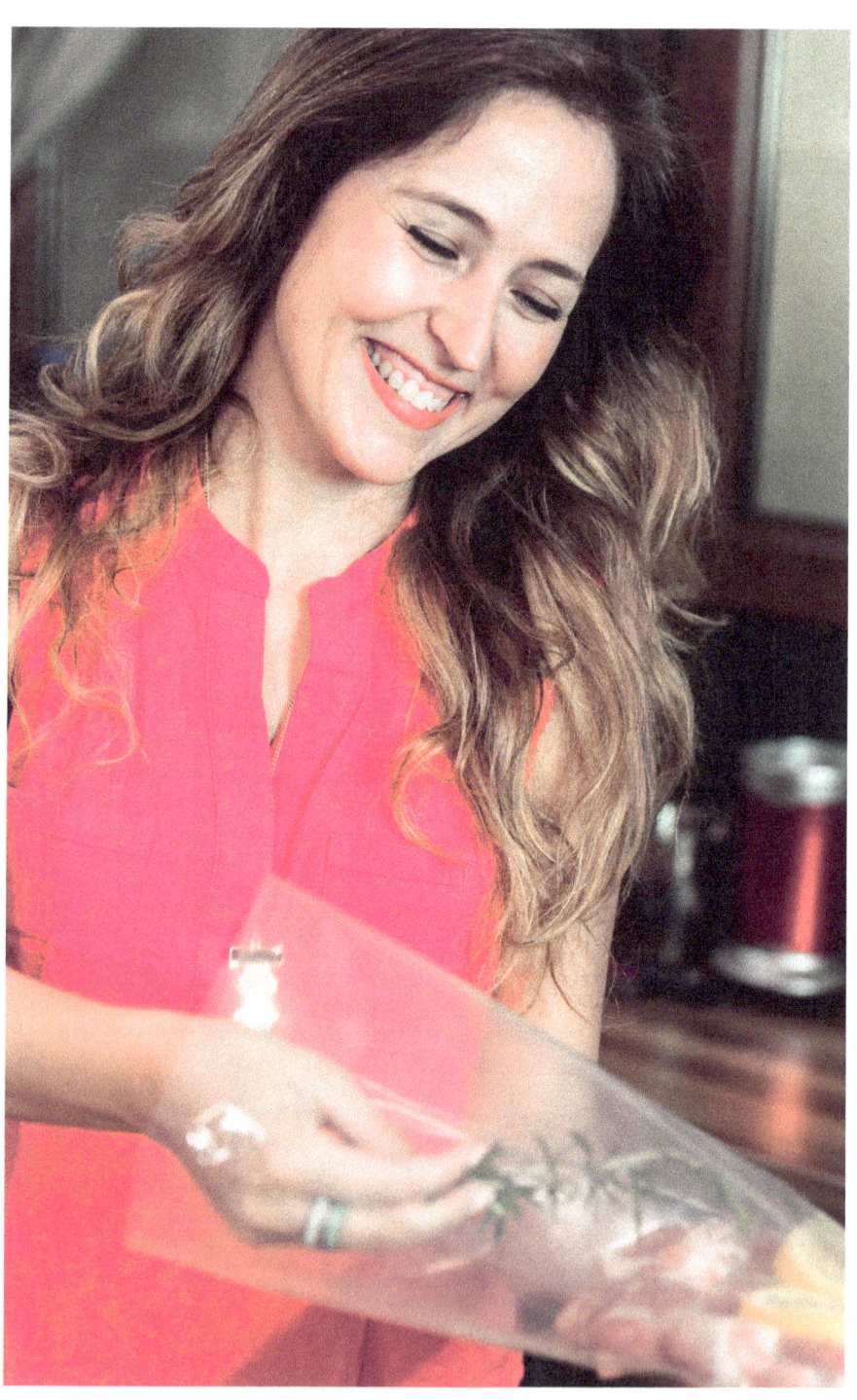

INTRODUCTION

Cooking is something that runs in my blood, most of my food memories are of my Nan cooking Sunday dinners - lasagna and cannelloni to share with the whole family. When I was young, I have never liked to be stuck in a classroom, I started culinary school at a very young age, and the only thing I really wanted was to be out cooking. You could say I was not a particularly good student, but I have always been really passionate about food.

I have been working in a professional kitchen since I was seventeen years old and I'm running my own restaurant since I was 23. The past thirty years have been a rewarding, yet arduous journey that I spent learning the basics and mastering the different cuisines and techniques by taking the best out of each of them. It was last year, during the lockdown, that I realized that I was starting to lose my passion. Preparing a dish had become an aseptic and mechanical where perfection was king.

I wanted to go back to my roots, cooking has always been about my family; preparing a dish together with the people I love gives me time to connect and create precious memories. Setting aside a time where the entire family can work together to create a meal gives us a chance to pause, catch up and just connect with each other.

What I would like to share with you in this book is my renewed passion and a technique that I learned during my time in France, the Sous Vide. This innovative cooking method is something my grandmother never thought existed and creates the perfect opportunity to spend some time in the kitchen with my family. For these reasons, I think the Sous Vide is the perfect combination of my professional and domestic life.

Sous Vide is the French term that translates to "under vacuum" and it is the method for preparing a dish at a specifically controlled temperature and time; your food should be prepared at the temperature at which it will be eaten. Put simply, this procedure involves placing food in vacuum seal bags and boiling it in a specially built bath of water for longer than average cooking times (usually 1 to 7 hours, up to 48 or more in some cases). Cooking at an exact temperature takes the guesswork out of the equation that defines a perfect meal. You can easily prepare your steak, chicken, lamb, pork, etc., exactly the way you like it, every single time.

It is easy to use and leads to great results every time. You will end up with food that is more tender and juicier than anything else you've ever made. This technique will help you to take your everyday cooking to a higher level. To do a top dish, most of the time, you do not need exotic ingredients, it is just a matter to get the best from the ingredients you already know.

The greatest part of Sous Vide cooking is that it does not require your constant presence in the kitchen. When the food is sealed in a bag and placed in the water bath, you can leave it at a low temperature, and it will cook on its own without asking much of your attention. The Sous Vide Cookers that are nowadays available in the market are efficient at regulating the perfect temperature to cook food according to its texture while maintaining the minimum required temperature. So, while your food is in the water, your hands are practically free to work on other important tasks or spend some quality time with your family.

It is an artful skill that is definitely worth trying. If it is just your first time, don't feel bad if you don't get the results you wanted to achieve. You will get better by gaining experience with this cookbook! The key is having patience, the right information, and consistency.

The meals prepared with Sous Vide are tasty and healthy, since this technique does not use added fats during the preparation of your dish also, using low temperature ensures that the perfect cooking point is reached.

Dishes included in this cookbook are simple, delicious, and provide you with so many options that you'll be preparing them for years to come. These recipes are made to be shared with the people you love and to build new precious food memories as I did with my Nan.

RECIPES

1. CRISPY EGG YOLKS

Cal.: 161 | Fat: 6.3g | Protein: 9.5g

Preparation Time: 11 minutes
Cooking Time: 65 minutes
Servings: 4

Ingredients

4 + 1 egg
4 tablespoons all-purpose flour
1/3 teaspoon baking powder
½ cup breadcrumbs
½ teaspoon fine salt
¾ teaspoon black truffle salt
Salt and pepper, to taste

Directions

1. Fill and preheat the cooker to 148°F/64°C.

2. Cook four eggs for 60 minutes. Let the eggs cool in cold water for 10 minutes.

3. Carefully peel the eggs, and let the egg white drip out.

4. Reserve egg yolks.

5. Heat 1-inch oil in a skillet over medium heat.

6. While the oil is heating, whisk flour, baking powder, and salt in a bowl.

7. Beat the remaining egg in a small bowl.

8. Dredge egg yolks in flour and dip into beaten egg. Finally, roll in breadcrumbs.

9. Fry in heated oil until golden brown.

10. Drain the egg yolks on a paper towel. Sprinkle with black truffle salt.

11. Serve.

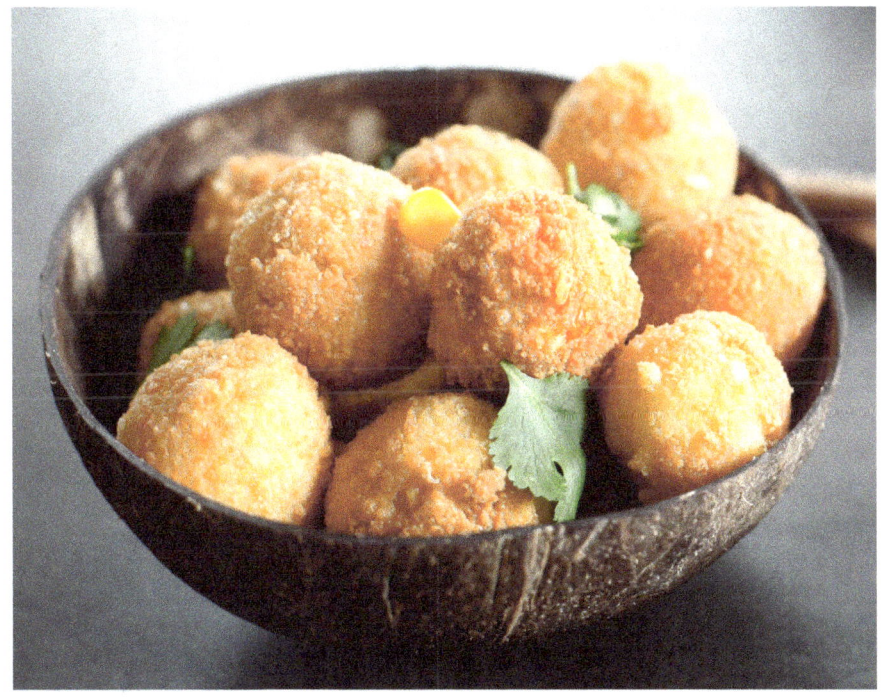

2. EGGS AND OREGANO

Cal.: 331 | Fat: 7g | Protein: 7g

Preparation Time: 9 minutes
Cooking Time: 32 minutes
Servings: 2

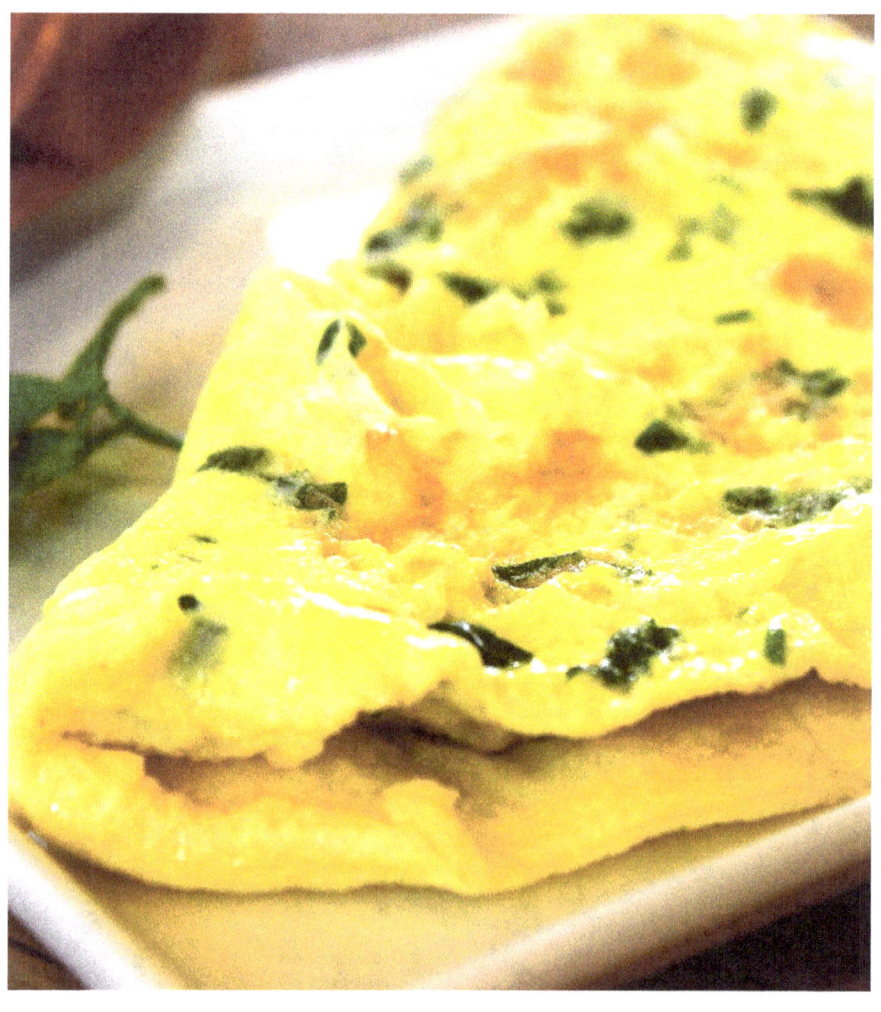

Ingredients

1 red bell pepper, chopped
2 shallots, chopped
4 eggs, whisked
A pinch of salt and black pepper
1 tablespoon oregano, chopped
½ teaspoon chili powder
½ teaspoon sweet paprika

Directions

1. Prepare your sous-vide water bath to a temperature of 170°F/76°C.

2. Pour the whisked egg into a cooking pouch and add the other ingredients.

3. Immerse the pouch into the water bath and cook for 30 minutes.

4. Once done, remove the pouch from the water bath and transfer the contents to a serving plate.

5. Serve and enjoy!

3. COCKTAIL MEATBALLS

Cal.: 276 | Fat: 18g | Protein: 24g

Preparation Time: 10 minutes
Cooking Time: 3 hours
Servings: 10

Ingredients

2 eggs
½ pound mild sausage, ground
½ cup seasoned breadcrumbs
1 pound ground beef
½ pound ground pork
1 cup leeks, finely chopped
1 teaspoon garlic paste
Salt and ground black pepper, to taste
½ teaspoon ancho chili powder
1 teaspoon dried basil
½ teaspoon dried marjoram
1/4 teaspoon ground allspice

Directions

1. Prepare your sous-vide water bath to a temperature of 146°F/63°C.

2. Add all the ingredients to a bowl and mix thoroughly.

3. Using your hand, shape the mixture into balls.

4. Put the balls into a cooking pouch and seal it after removing the excess air.

5. Immerse the pouch into the water bath.

6. Cook for 3 hours.

7. Grease a nonstick pan with cooking spray.

8. Sear the meatballs in batches. Sear each side for 3 minutes.

9. Serve and enjoy!

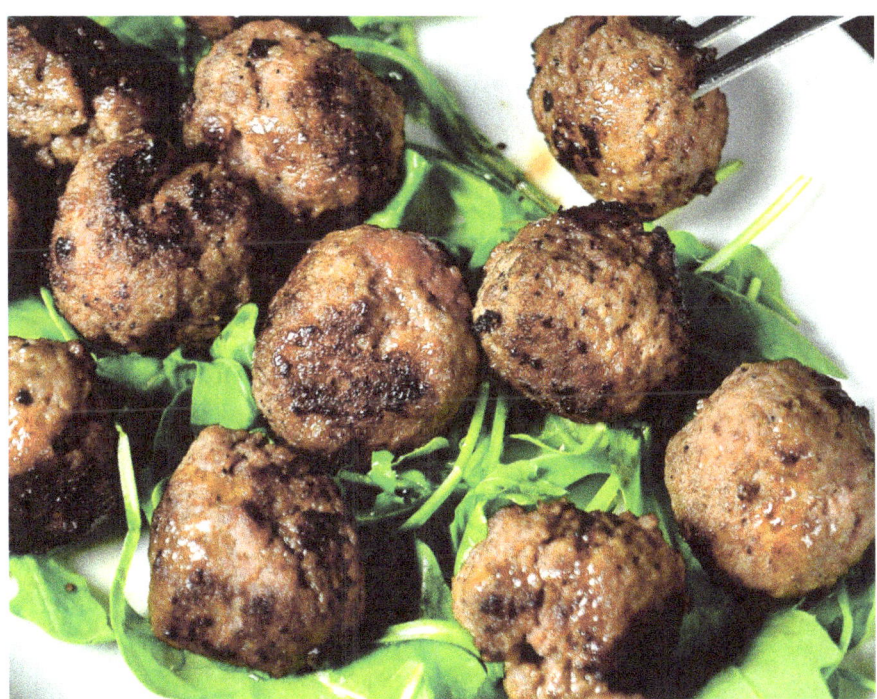

4. WHITE BEAN AND ARTICHOKE DIP

Cal.: 304 | Fat: 20g | Protein: 13g

Preparation Time: 10 minutes
Cooking Time: 4 hours
Servings: 6

Ingredients

½ cup dried cannellini beans
1½ cups water
2 garlic cloves, divided.
1 (14-ounce) can artichoke hearts, drained
2 tablespoons lemon juice
2 tablespoons extra-virgin olive oil
½ teaspoon sea salt
1/3 cup grated Parmesan cheese.

Directions

1. Fill the water bath with water. Set your machine temperature to 195°F/91°C.

2. Place the beans, 1½ cups water, and 1 garlic clove in a large food-safe zip-top bag. Slowly lower the zip-top bag into the water and, using the water displacement method, the air will escape from the bag. Continue to lower the bag until it is about 1"

from being fully Immersed. Once the bag has been lowered, zip it shut with your fingers.

3. Cook for 3 ½ hours. Check to see if the beans are tender and cook a little longer if needed.

4. Drain the beans and let them cool until they come to room temperature.

5. Using a food processor, pulse the beans, artichoke hearts, lemon juice, remaining garlic clove, oil, salt and Parmesan cheese. Process until smooth and creamy. If a thinner consistency is desired, add a little extra water while processing. Serve.

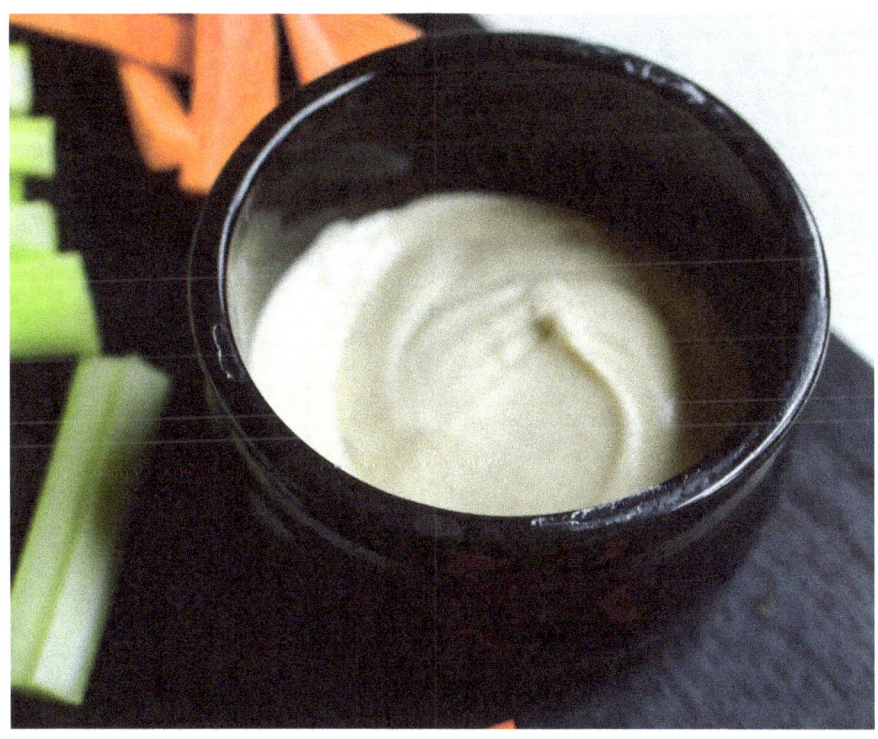

5. SALTY CUSTARD

Cal.: 168 | Fat: 12.5g | Protein: 12.9g

Preparation Time: 11 minutes
Cooking Time: 30 minutes
Servings: 4

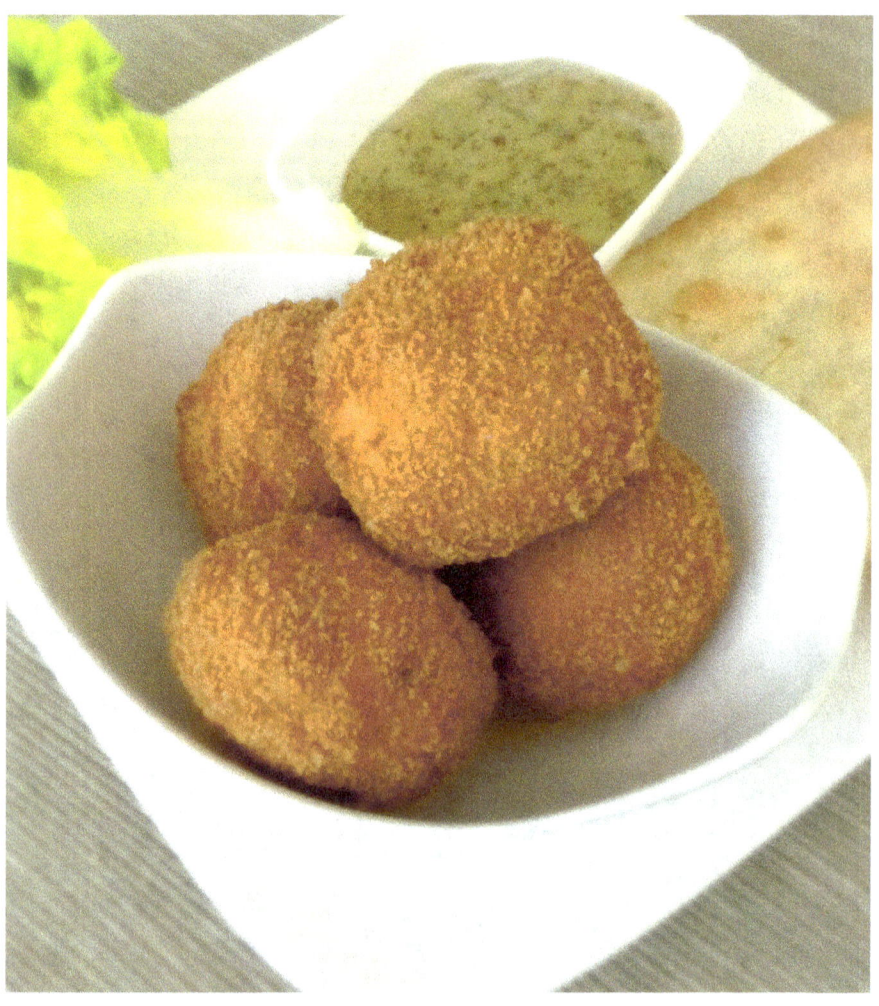

Ingredients

8 large eggs
2 cups chicken stock
2 teaspoons sesame oil
Salt and pepper, to taste
Soy sauce, chopped green onion

Directions

1. Fill and preheat the sous-vide cooker to 180°F/82°C.

2. In a blender, blend eggs, chicken stock, sesame oil, salt, and pepper until smooth.

3. Strain through a fine-mesh sieve to remove any foam.

4. If needed, strain again and transfer into the vacuum bag. Seal the bag and immerse into the water bath.

5. Cook for 20 minutes. Remove from the water bath and shake or massage gently.

6. Cook 10 minutes additional. Remove from the water bath and place into an ice-cold bath for 20 minutes.

7. Serve in a bowl, and top with a splash of soy sauce and chopped green onion.

6. SPRING ONION SOUP

Cal.: 368 | Fat: 28g | Protein: 10g

Preparation Time: 14 minutes
Cooking Time: 1 hour
Servings: 2

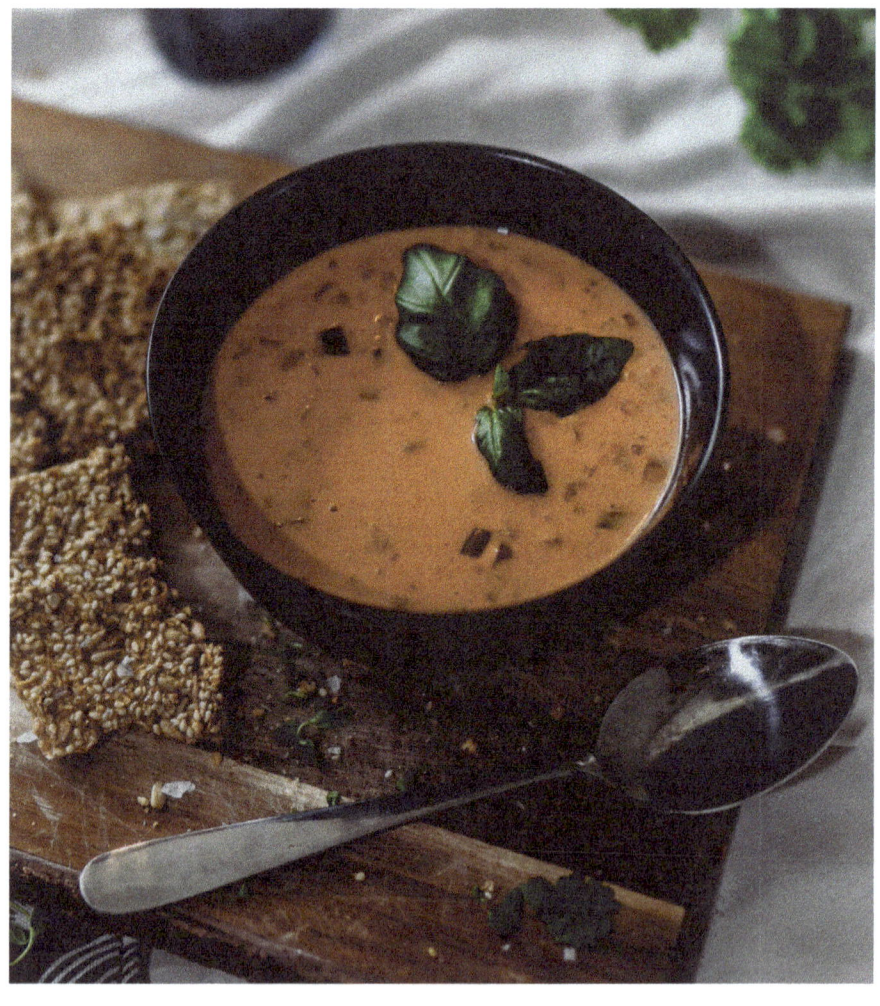

Ingredients

2 bunches of spring onions, rinsed, trimmed, chopped
4 garlic cloves, peeled, chopped
1 large russet potato, peeled, diced
2 teaspoons olive oil plus extra for serving
2 teaspoons soy sauce
Salt to taste
Pepper powder to taste
2-3 tablespoons fresh parsley leaves for garnishing

Directions

1. Set your Sous Vide machine to 180°F/82°C.

2. Add all the ingredients into a ziplock or a vacuum-seal bag and remove all the air. Seal and immerse the bag in the water bath and cook for 45 minutes to 1 hour.

3. Remove the pouch and transfer into a blender and blend until smooth and creamy.

4. Ladle into individual soup bowls. Garnish with parsley and serve.

7. SPRING MINESTRONE SOUP

Cal.: 330 | Fat: 7g | Protein: 7g

Preparation Time: 10 minutes
Cooking Time: 40 minutes
Servings: 4

Ingredients

2 chopped carrots
1 sliced leek
Sprigs thyme
3 chopped red potatoes
2 tablespoons olive oil
Cups vegetable broth
1 bunch sliced asparagus
2 cups navy beans
2 tablespoons chopped dill
Salt

Directions

1. Take a large mixing pan and combine the carrots, thyme, leek and salt.

2. Preheat the Sous Vide machine to 165°F/74°C.

3. Take the above mixture in a Ziploc bag and seal it.

4. Place the bag in and cook for 8 minutes.

5. Take a large skillet and take the cooked vegetables, add red potatoes, vegetable broth and cook for 25 minutes until they turn tender.

6. Then add asparagus and cook for 3 more minutes. Remove thyme and add navy beans, chopped dill, salt and pepper.

7. Serve hot.

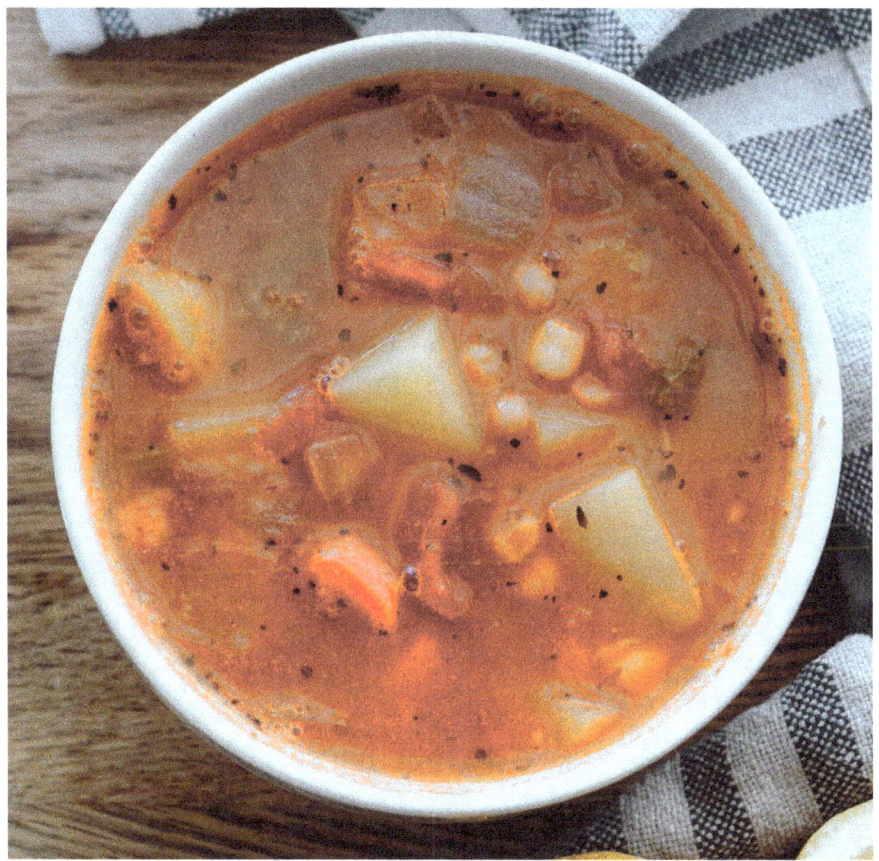

8. MUSHROOM ORZO GREEN SOUP

Cal.: 230 | Fat: 7g | Protein: 8g

Preparation Time: 5 minutes
Cooking Time: 35 minutes
Servings: 6

Ingredients

1 cup sliced mushroom
1 cup orzo
3 cups sliced spinach
3 cups broccoli
Cups vegetable broth
2 tablespoons olive oil
1 1/4 cup celery
½ cup shallots
1/4 cup garlic
Salt, pepper and basil pesto

Directions

1. In a large cooking pan mix the celery, shallots, garlic, salt and oil.

2. Preheat the Sous Vide machine to 175°F/79°C.

3. Take the above mix in a Ziploc pouch. Seal it under

vacuum or under water.

4. Place the bag in and cook for 8 minutes.

5. Take the cooked vegetables in a skillet and add vegetable broth and broccoli. Simmer for 15 minutes.

6. Add mushroom, orzo, spinach and simmer again for 10 minutes until all vegetables soften.

7. Sprinkle salt, pepper, basil pesto and serve hot.

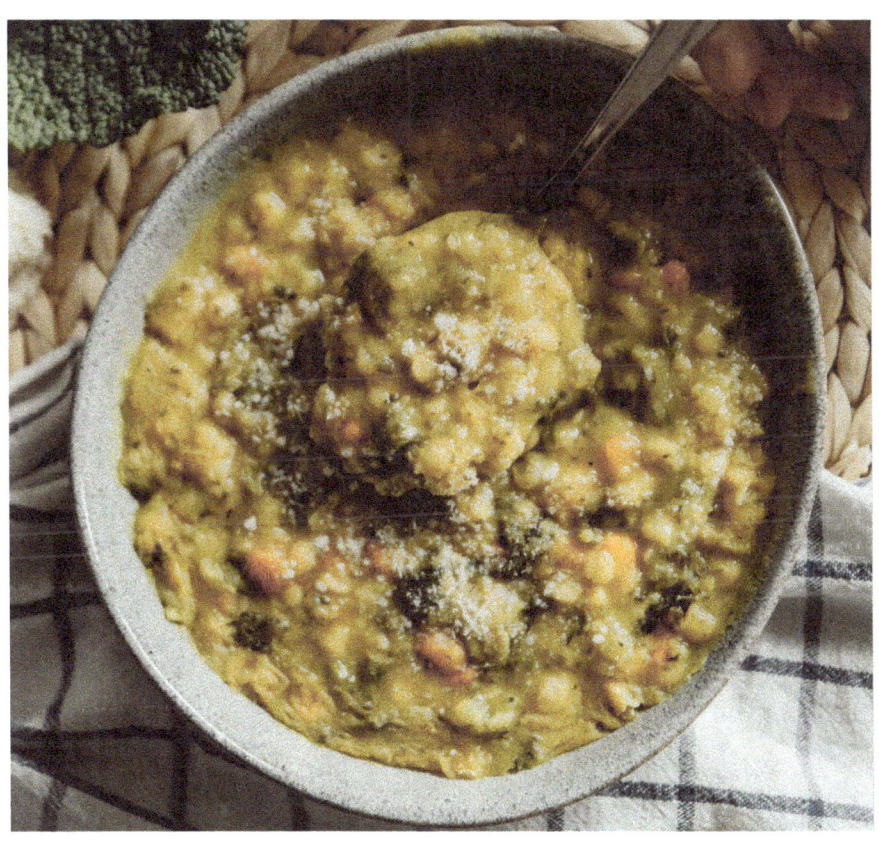

9. POTATO AND CURRY SOUP

Cal.: 355 | Fat: 11g | Protein: 17g

Preparation Time: 10 minutes
Cooking Time: 1 hour
Servings: 4

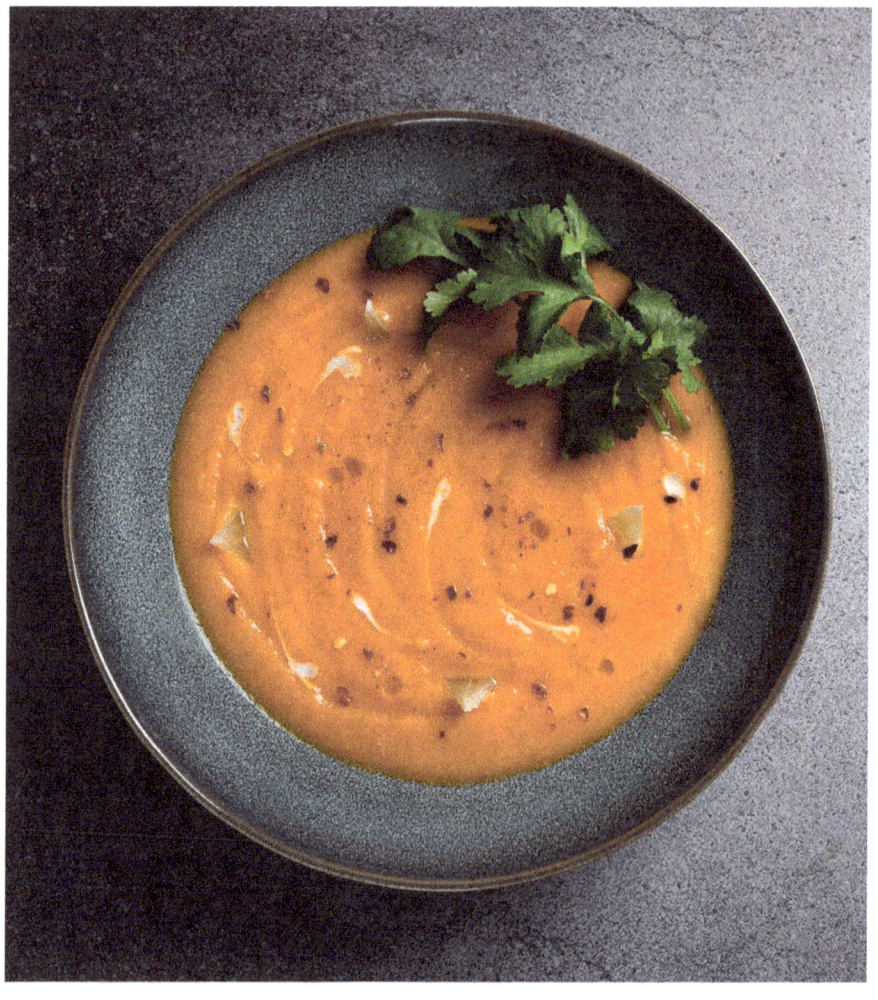

Ingredients

1 onion, chopped
2 garlic cloves, minced
1 carrot, peeled and grated
1 ½ cup potato, peeled and cubed
2 cups vegetable stock
Salt and pepper to taste
2 tbsp. curry powder
Chopped cilantro for serving

Directions

1. Preheat the Sous Vide machine to 183°F/84°C.

2. Put the vegetables and curry powder into the vacuum bag, and seal it, removing the air.

3. Set the cooking time for 50 minutes.

4. Transfer the cooked vegetables to a pot, add the vegetable stock and blend everything together using an immersion blender.

5. Bring the soup to a boil and simmer for 2–3 minutes.

6. Add salt and pepper to taste.

7. Serve with vegan yogurt and chopped dill or cilantro.

10. BOURBON CHICKEN

Cal.: 566 | Fat: 23.9g | Protein: 67.2g

Preparation Time: 20 minutes
Cooking Time: 1 hour 10 minutes
Servings: 4

Ingredients

2 pounds boneless chicken breasts, cut into bite-size pieces
2 tablespoons olive oil
1 garlic clove, crushed
1/4 teaspoon ginger
3/4 teaspoons crushed red pepper flakes
1/4 cup apple juice
1/3 cup light brown sugar
2 tablespoons ketchup
1 tablespoon cider vinegar
½ cup water
1/3 cup soy sauce

Directions

1. Set your immersion circulator to 150°F/65.5°C.

2. In a medium pan, heat the oil until hot but not smoking. Add the chicken and cook just until lightly browned. Remove chicken from heat.

3. Add the remaining ingredients and chicken to a vacuum-sealed bag.

4. Place the bag into the water bath and cook for one hour. This will give the ingredients time to combine into a flavorful sauce and finish cooking the chicken.

5. Remove the bag from the water bath and serve with steamed white or brown rice, or your choice of vegetables that can be cooked in a separate bag at the same time.

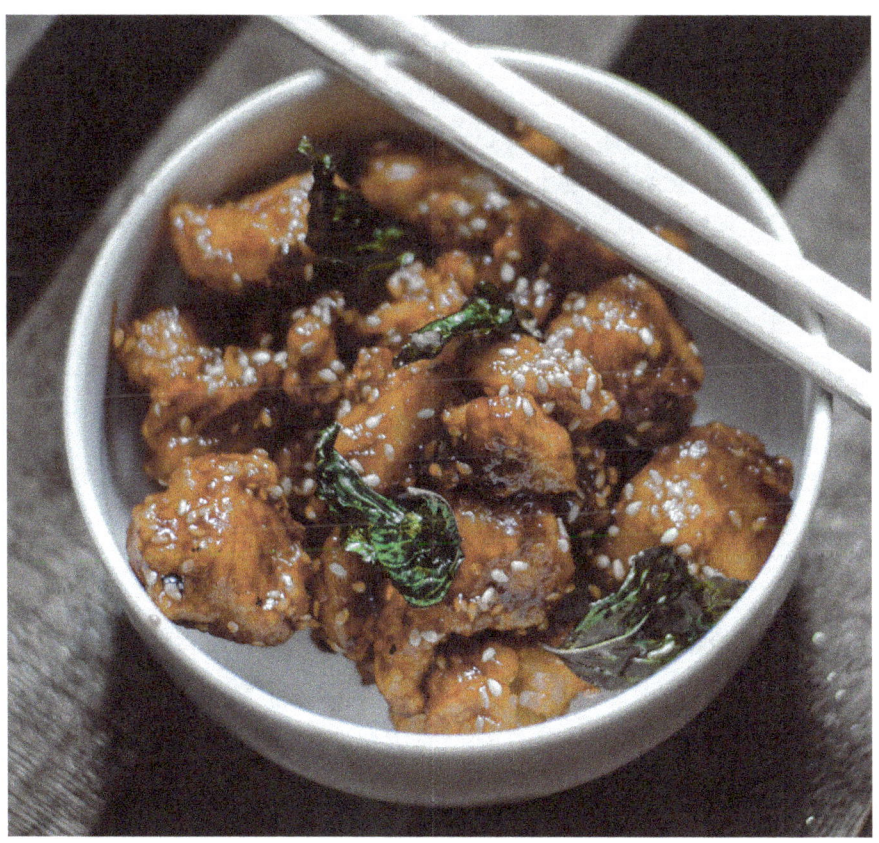

11. LEMON HERB TURKEY BREAST

Cal.: 639 | Fat: 7.9g | Protein: 78.8g

Preparation Time: 6 minutes
Cooking Time: 4 hours
Servings: 2

Ingredients

2 lbs. boneless, skinless turkey breast
1/4 cup honey
1/4 cup lemon juice
1 teaspoon dried dill or 1 tablespoon fresh
1 teaspoon dried parsley or 1 tablespoon fresh
1 teaspoon dried basil or 1 tablespoon fresh
1/4 teaspoon black pepper
1 teaspoon salt
2 tablespoons flour

Directions

1. Preheat the Sous Vide machine to 143°F/62°C.

2. Combine all the ingredients except for the turkey and flour in a bowl. Place the turkey in the bag along with the marinade mixture. Seal the bag and place in the water bath. Cook for 4 hours.

3. When the turkey is cooked, put the flour in a small saucepan along with 1 tablespoon oil. Heat the mixture over medium heat, stirring constantly for about 1 minute. Pour in the juices from the bag and use a whisk to remove any lumps from the gravy.

4. Slice the turkey thin and serve with the gravy.

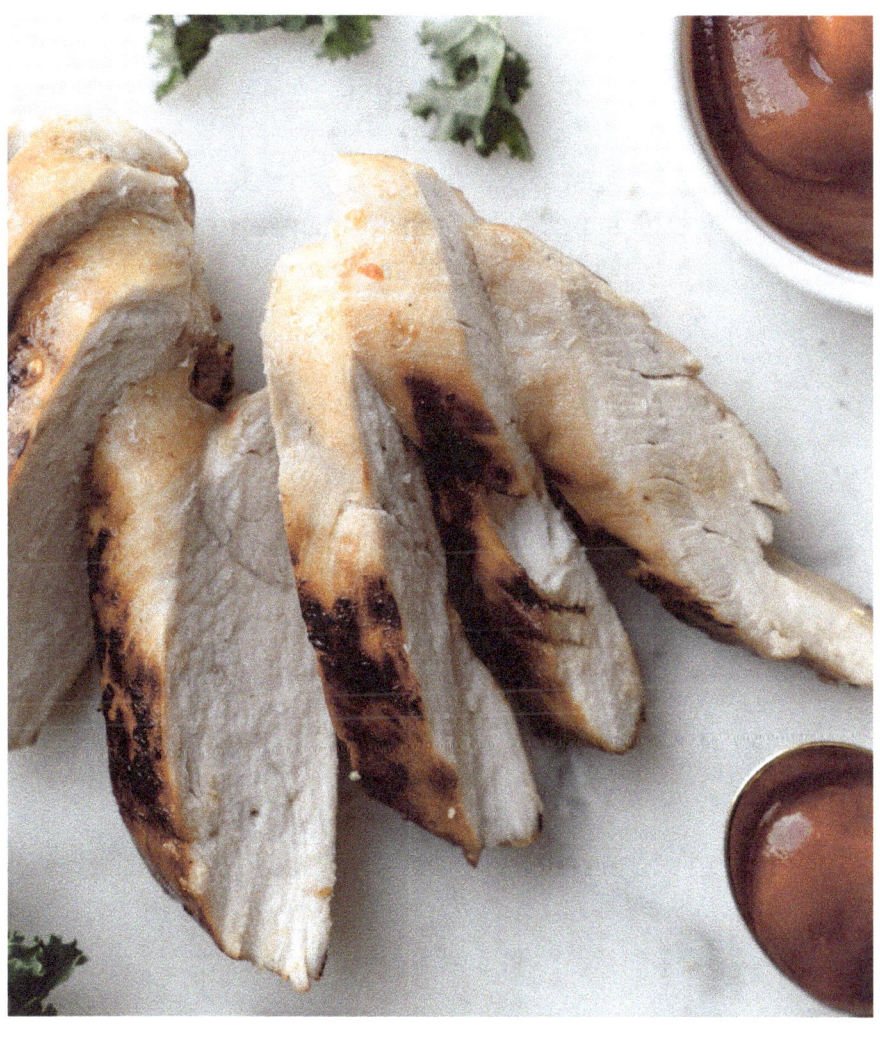

12. ARROWROOT COUNTRY-STYLE RIBS

Cal.: 280 | Fat: 9g | Protein: 42g

Preparation Time: 26 minutes
Cooking Time: 18 hours
Servings: 10

Ingredients

1 teaspoon mustard powder
1 cup stock, preferably homemade
1/3 cup tamari sauce
4 pounds country-style ribs
½ teaspoon onion powder
½ teaspoon garlic powder
½ teaspoon ground ginger
2 tablespoons arrowroot powder
½ cup brown sugar, packed

Directions

1. Prepare your Sous-vide water bath to a temperature of 145°F/63°C.

2. Put the stock, ribs, mustard powder, garlic and onion powder into a Ziploc bag and seal it after squeezing out the excess air.

3. Immerse the bag into the water bath and cook for 18 hours.

4. Preheat your oven to 360°F/182°C.

5. Put the ribs and the cooking liquid in a baking pan.

6. Get a bowl and add the tamari, arrowroot, sugar and ground pepper.

7. Mix the sauce and drizzle it over the ribs.

8. Bake the ribs for 20 minutes until crispy.

9. Serve and enjoy!

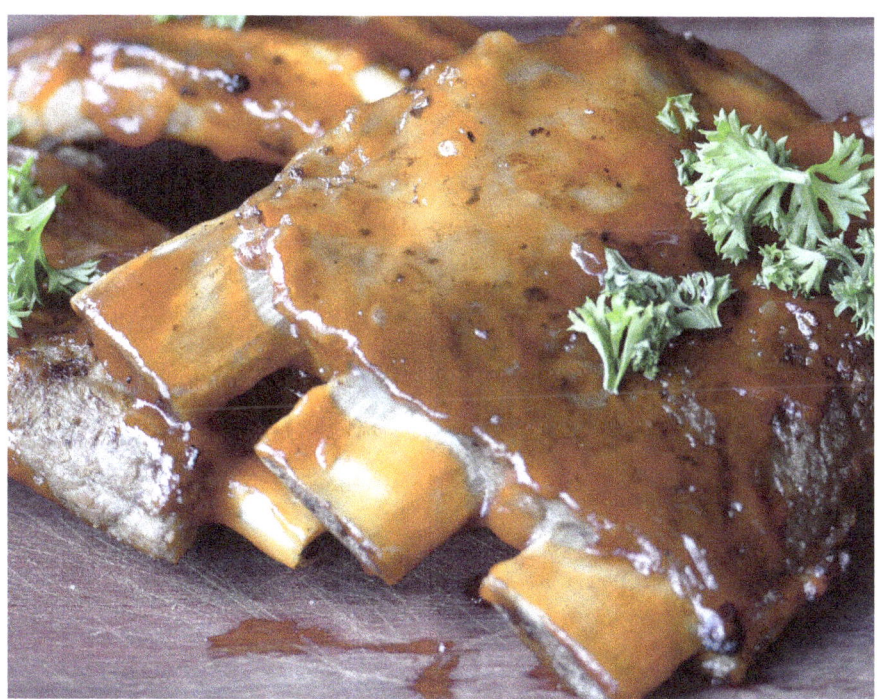

13. BEEF TRI-TIP WITH BBQ SAUCE

Cal.: 163 | Fat: 5.6g | Protein: 18.2g

Preparation Time: 11 minutes
Cooking Time: 6 hours
Servings: 6

Ingredients

2 ½ lb. beef tri-tip
2 teaspoons kosher salt
1 teaspoon freshly ground black pepper
½ cup barbecue sauce, divided
2 teaspoons light brown sugar

Directions

1. Preheat the Sous Vide machine to 130°F/55°C.

2. Season beef with 1 teaspoon salt and ½ teaspoon black pepper.

3. Transfer meat to a Ziploc bag and add ¼ cup barbecue sauce.

4. Seal the bag using the water immersion technique and place in a water bath for 6 hours.

5. When the timer goes off, remove the bag from the water bath.

6. Take out the meat and pat dry with kitchen towels.

7. Preheat the broiler to medium heat and place the meat on the foil-lined broiler-safe baking sheet.

8. Brush the meat with remaining sauce and sprinkle with sugar, remaining salt and pepper.

9. Broil for 5 minutes or until caramelized.

10. Place the meat on the serving platter and let it rest for 10 minutes.

11. Slice before serving.

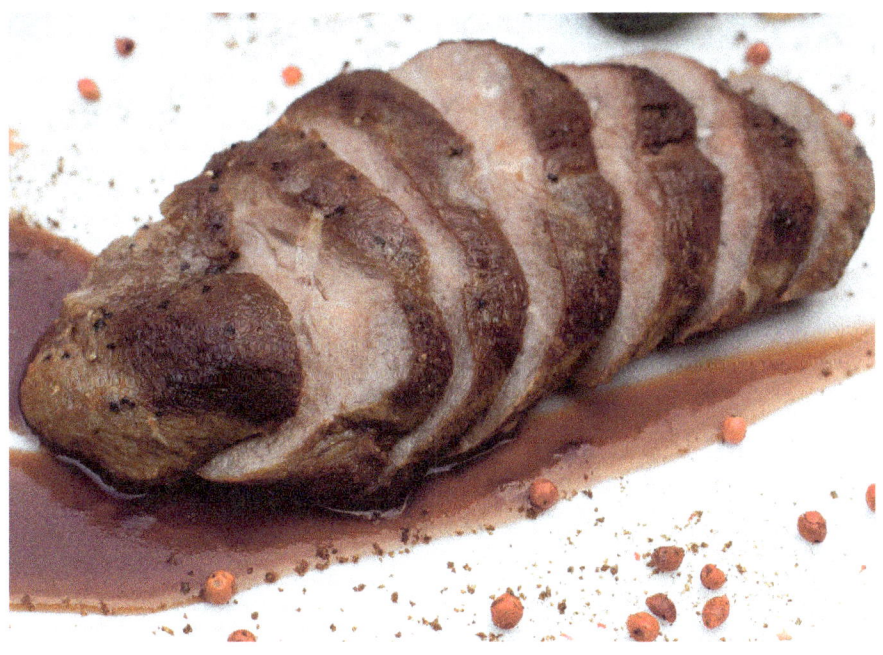

14. HERB RUB PORK CHOPS

Cal.: 383 | Fat: 33.1g | Protein: 18.6g

Preparation Time: 10 minutes
Cooking Time: 2 hours 10 minutes
Servings: 4

Ingredients

4 pork chops, bone-in
1/4 cup olive oil
1 tsp. black pepper
1 tbsp. balsamic vinegar
1 lemon zest
2 garlic cloves, minced
6 thyme sprigs, remove stems
1/4 cup chives
1/4 cup rosemary
10 basil leaves
1/4 cup parsley
½ tsp. salt

Directions

1. Preheat the Sous Vide machine to 140 F/ 60 C.

2. Add herbs to the food processor and process until chopped.

3. Add garlic, olive oil, pepper, salt, vinegar, and lemon zest and blend until a smooth paste.

4. Rub herb mixture over pork chops. Place pork chops into the Ziploc bag and remove all the air from the bag before sealing.

5. Place the bag into the hot water bath and cook for 2 hours.

6. Remove pork chops from the water bath and boil for 3-4 minutes.

7. Serve and enjoy!

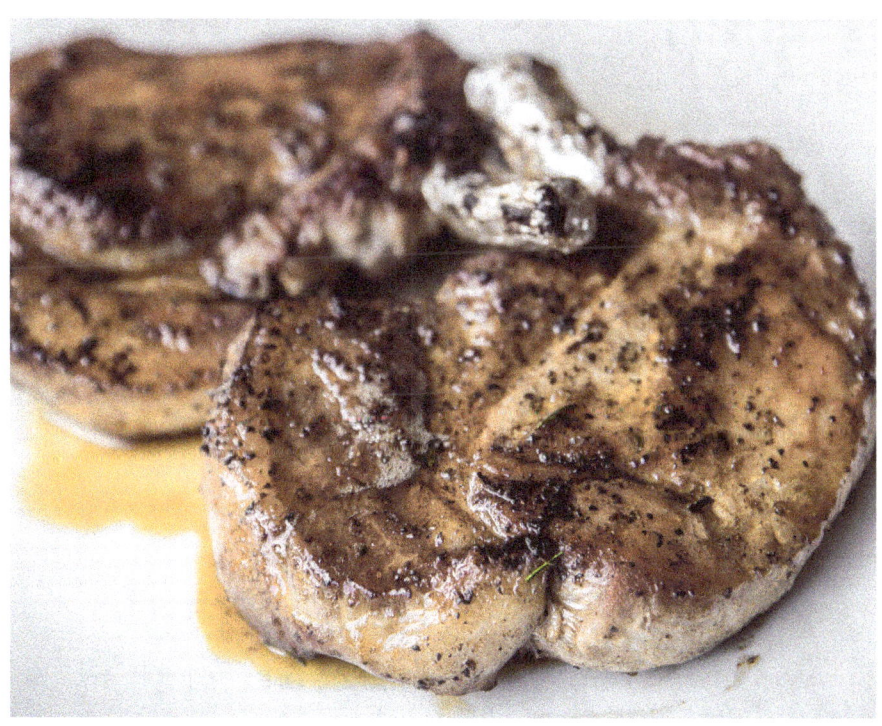

15. CHOPPED DUCK WITH HONEY

Cal.: 229 | Fat: 13.3g | Protein: 15g

Preparation Time: 18 minutes
Cooking Time: 4 hours
Servings: 6

Ingredients

4 tablespoon liquid honey
1 teaspoon nutmeg
1 tablespoon ground paprika
18 oz. duck fillet
1 teaspoon ground cinnamon
1 teaspoon fresh dill

Directions

1. Pour the liquid honey into the plastic bag.

2. Add the nutmeg and ground paprika.

3. Then add the ground cinnamon and fresh dill.

4. Close the plastic bag and massage it to make the homogenous mixture.

5. After this, chop the duck fillet and add it to the

plastic bag too.

6. Close the plastic bag again and massage it with the help of the fingers to make the homogenous meat mixture.

7. Leave the chopped duck mixture for 10 minutes to marinate.

8. After this, preheat the water bath to 147°F/64°C.

9. Seal the plastic bag with the chopped duck and put it in the water bath.

10. Cook the chopped duck for 4 hours.

11. When the dish is cooked, transfer it directly to the serving plates.

12. Enjoy the dish immediately!

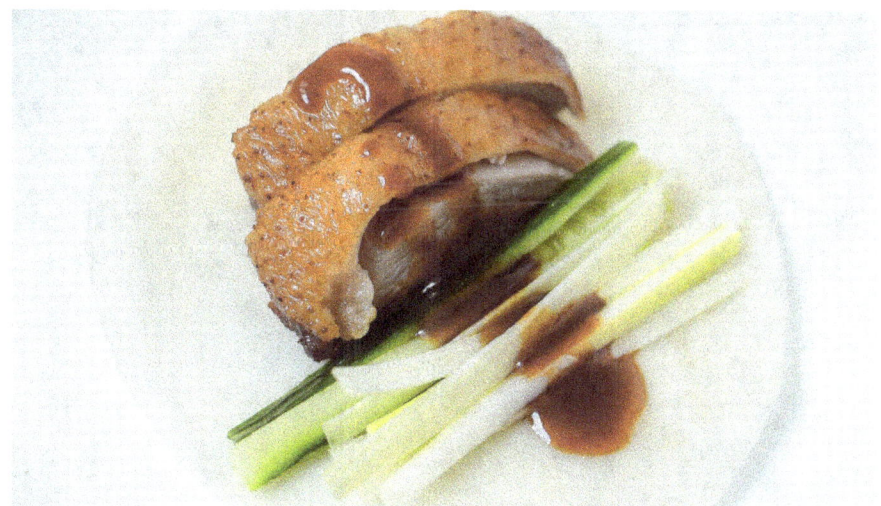

16. BBQ PORK RIBS

Cal.: 663 | Fat: 19g | Protein: 10g

Preparation Time: 5 minutes
Cooking Time: 18 hours
Servings: 2

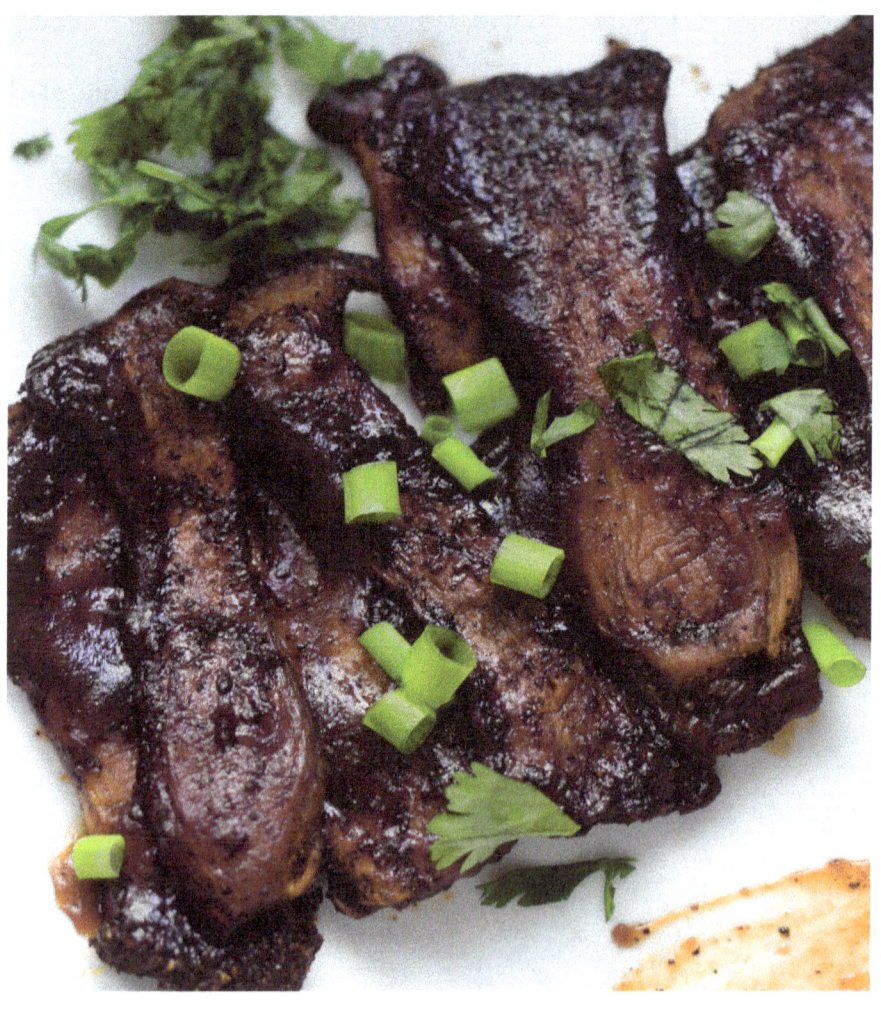

Ingredients

1 rack back ribs, cut into rib portions
2 tbsp. Worcestershire sauce
1/3 cup brown sugar
1 ½ cups BBQ sauce

Directions

1. Preheat the Sous Vide machine to 160°F/75°C.

2. Whisk brown sugar in 1 cup BBQ sauce and Worcestershire sauce.

3. Place ribs into the large mixing bowl then pour marinade over ribs and toss well.

4. Place ribs into the Ziploc bag and remove all the air from the bag before sealing.

5. Place the bag into the hot water bath and cook for 18 hours.

6. Remove ribs from the bag and place on a baking tray.

7. Brush ribs with remaining BBQ sauce and broil for 5 minutes.

8. Serve and enjoy!

17. SIMPLE SLICED PORK BELLY

Cal.: 374 | Fat: 25g | Protein: 27g

Preparation Time: 10 minutes
Cooking Time: 3 hours 10 minutes
Servings: 2

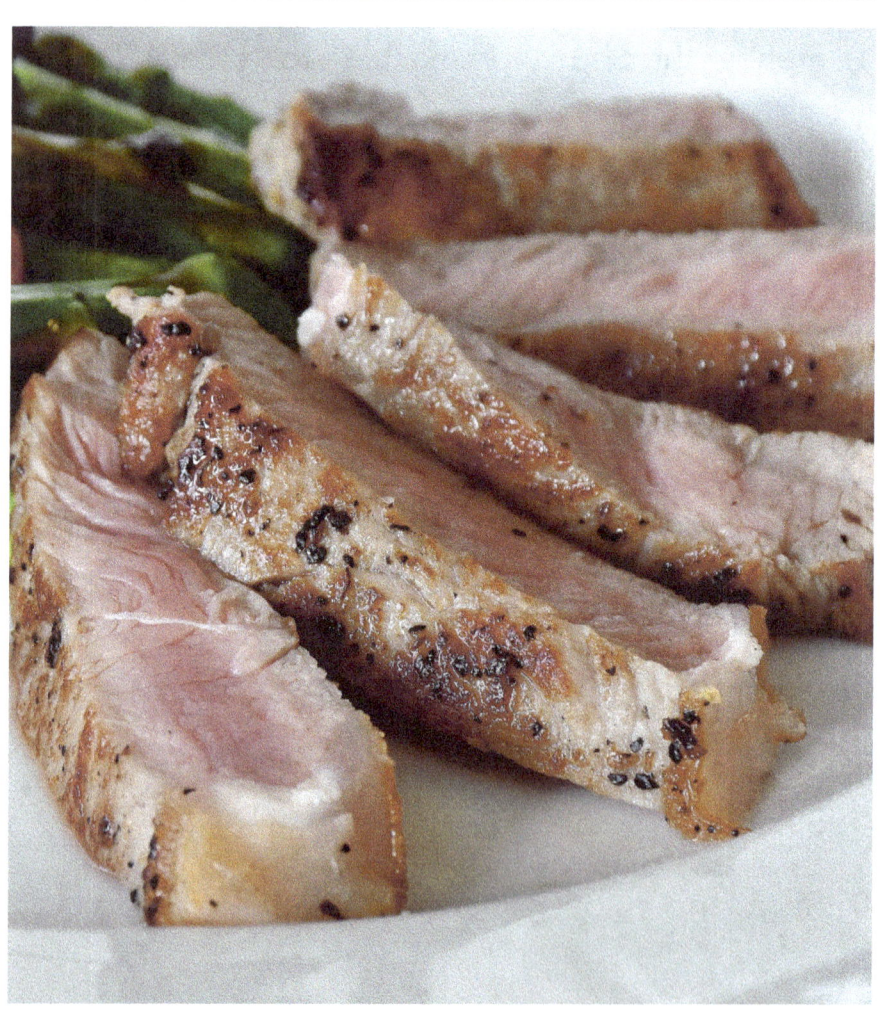

Ingredients

4 oz. pork belly, sliced
3 bay leaves
1 tbsp. garlic salt
1 tbsp. whole black peppercorns
1 ½ tbsp. olive oil

Directions

1. Preheat the Sous Vide machine to 145°F/62°C.

2. Add sliced pork belly, bay leaves, garlic salt, peppercorns, and 1 tbsp. of olive oil into the large Ziploc bag.

3. Remove all the air from the bag before sealing.

4. Place the bag into the hot water bath and cook for 3 hours.

5. Heat remaining oil in a pan over medium heat.

6. Remove pork from bag and sear in hot oil for 2 minutes on each side.

7. Serve and enjoy!

18. ROSEMARY GARLIC LAMB CHOPS

Cal.: 349 | Fat: 29g | Protein: 19.2g

Preparation Time: 5 minutes
Cooking Time: 2 hours 30 minutes
Servings: 4

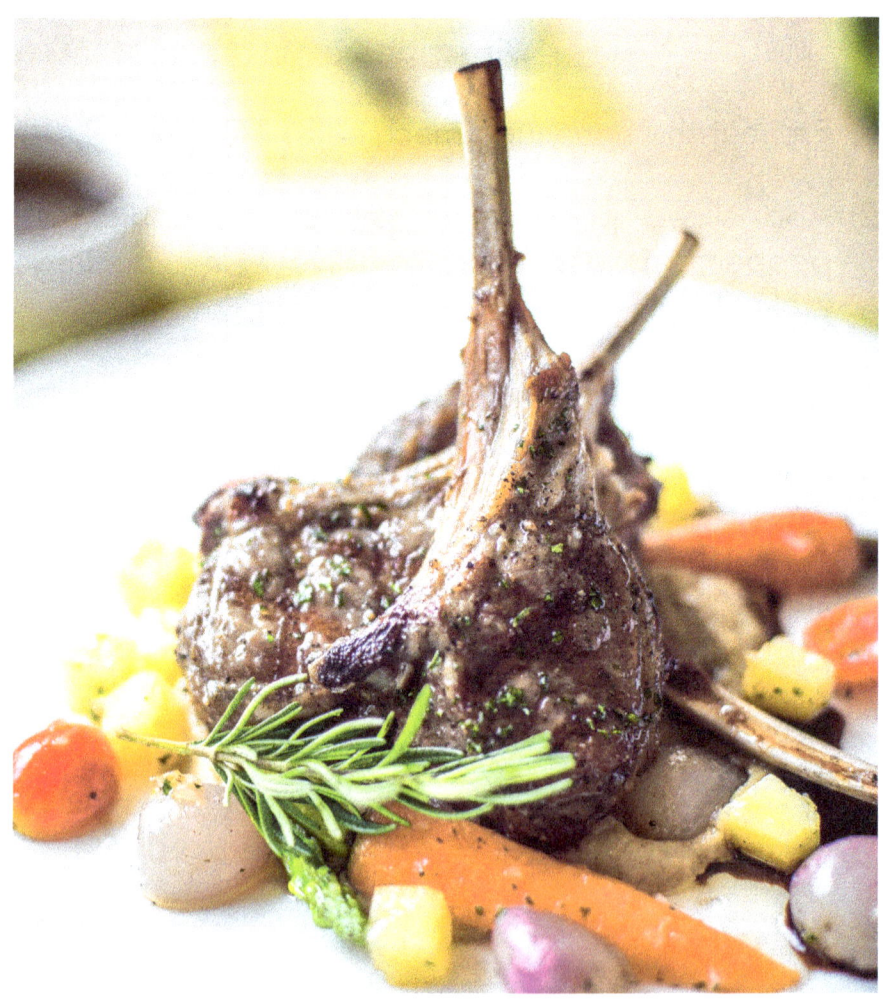

Ingredients

4 lamb chops
1 tbsp. butter
1 tsp. fresh thyme
1 tsp. fresh rosemary
2 garlic cloves
Pepper
Salt

Directions

1. Preheat the Sous Vide machine to 140°F/60°C.

2. Season lamb chops with pepper and salt.

3. Sprinkle lamb chops with garlic, thyme and rosemary.

4. Add butter to the Ziploc bag then place lamb chops into the bag.

5. Remove all air from the bag before sealing.

6. Place the bag in a hot water bath and cook for 2 ½ hours.

7. Once it's done, sear it on high heat until lightly brown. Serve and enjoy!

19. BACON

Cal.: 568 | Fat: 36.1g | Protein: 57g

Preparation Time: 11 minutes
Cooking Time: 8 hours
Servings: 4

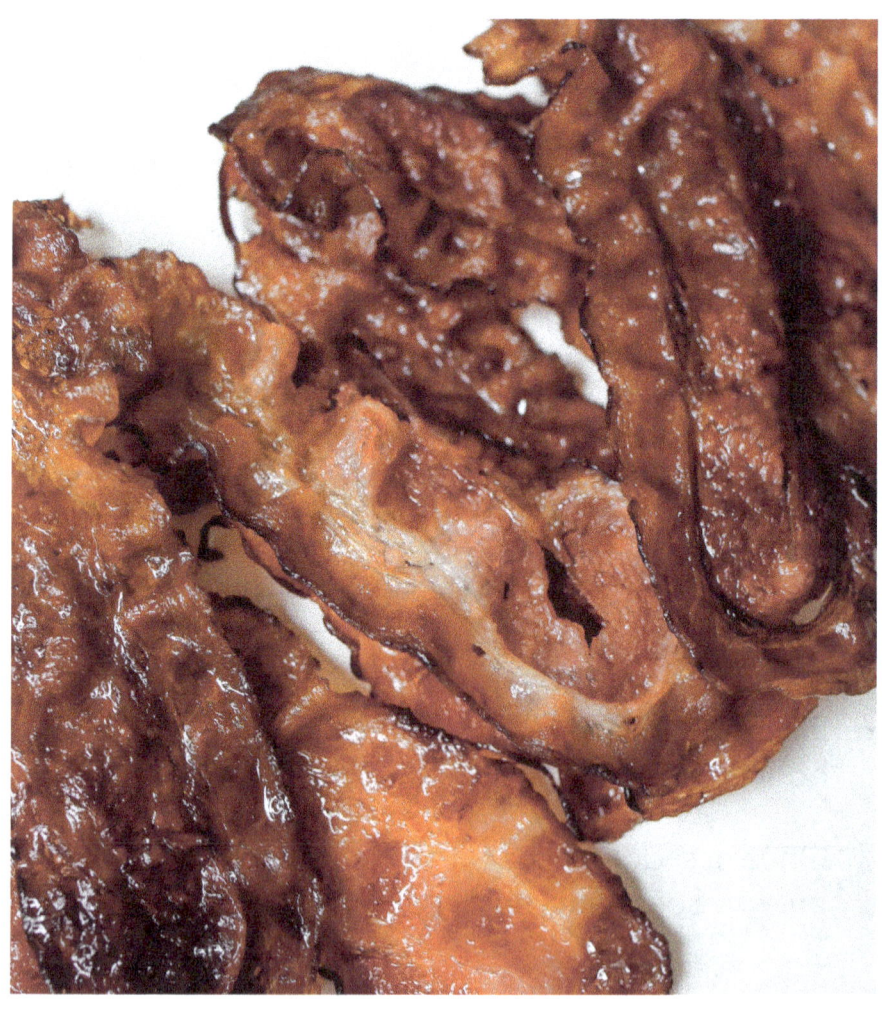

Ingredients

1 lb. pork bacon

Directions

1. Preheat the Sous Vide machine to 145°F/63°C.

2. Place the bacon in the bag you're going to use to sous and seal the bag.

3. Place the bag in the preheated water and set the timer for 8 hours.

4. When the bacon is almost done, heat a skillet on medium-high heat for a minimum of 5 minutes.

5. Place the bacon in the skillet and press down on it with a spatula to ensure it stays flat. Cook the bacon for around 2 minutes, until the bacon browns and becomes crispy. Then flip the bacon and cook it for an additional 15 seconds.

6. Place the bacon on a plate that has been lined with paper towels. Allow the excess grease to drain.

7. Serve while still hot.

20. TEMPTING TERIYAKI CHICKEN

Cal.: 300 | Fat: 4.1g | Protein: 27.1g

Preparation Time: 6 minutes
Cooking Time: 2 hours
Servings: 1

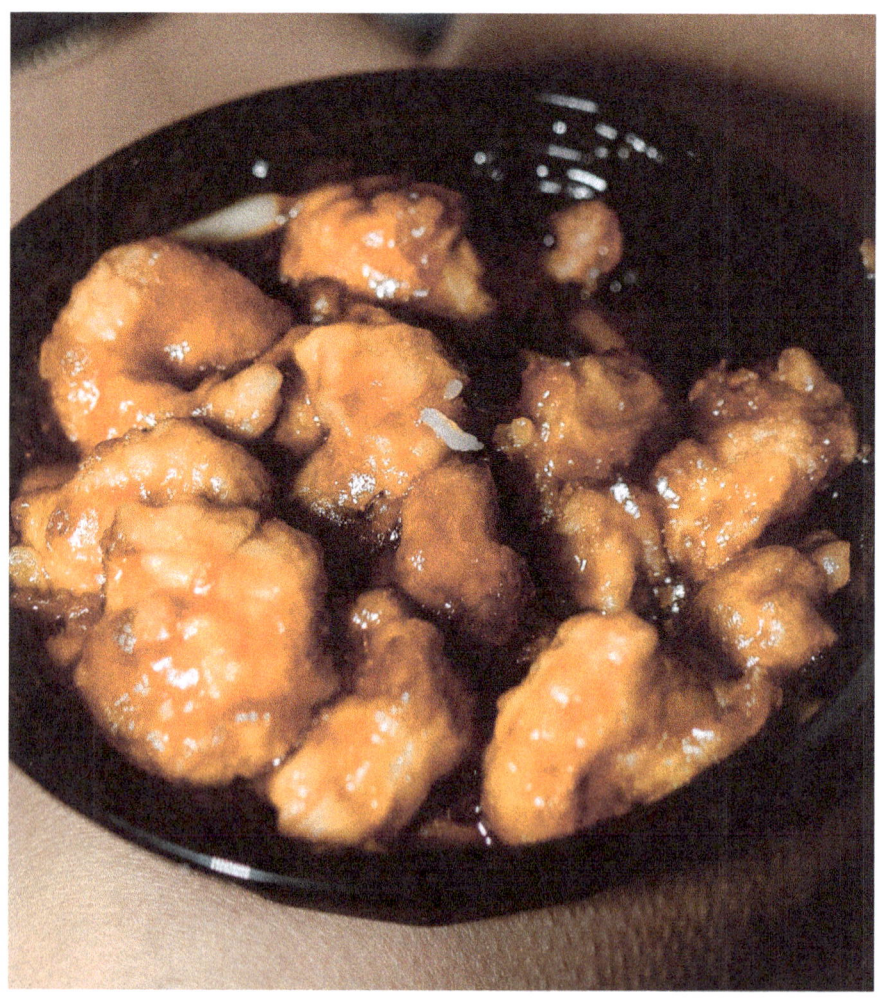

Ingredients

1 skinless, boneless chicken breast
½ teaspoon ginger juice
2 tablespoons sugar, plus 1 teaspoon
½ teaspoon salt
2 tablespoons soy sauce
2 tablespoons sake or mirin

Directions

1. Dry the chicken with a paper towel and then coat with ginger juice.

2. Mix 1 teaspoon sugar and salt in a small bowl, and sprinkle on both sides of the chicken.

3. Add the chicken to a vacuum bag and seal; set aside to marinate for 30 minutes or overnight.

4. Preheat water bath to 140°F/60°CAdd chicken and cook for 1 hour 30 minutes.

5. Combine the remaining sugar, soy sauce and sake in a small saucepan, bring to a boil, and cook until the sauce is thick, forming large shiny bubbles.

6. Remove sauce and place on warm until the chicken is done. Plate chicken, top with teriyaki sauce, and serve!

21. SPICED LAMB KEBABS

Cal.: 667 | Fat: 27.7g | Protein: 92.8g

Preparation Time: 16 minutes
Cooking Time: 2 hours
Servings: 4

Ingredients

2 garlic cloves, minced
Sea salt
Freshly ground black pepper
1 teaspoon dried oregano
1 tablespoon olive oil
4 lamb steaks cut into 2-inch chunks
2 red peppers, deseeded and cut into chunks
1 large onion, cut into chunks
2 lemons, cut into wedges
6 steel or bamboo skewers

Directions

1. Set your Sous Vide Machine to 140°F/60°C.

2. In a large bowl, combine the garlic, salt, pepper, oregano, olive oil and lamb chunks. Stir thoroughly to coat.

3. Spoon the lamb into a vacuum-sealed bag.

4. Immerse in the water bath and cook for 1-½ hours.

5. When the lamb is almost finished cooking, heat your oven to 500°F/260°C.

6. Remove the bag from the water and pat lamb dry with a paper towel.

7. Skewer the lamb, alternating lamb, pepper and onion chunks.

8. Arrange the skewers on a baking sheet and cook in the oven for 5 minutes. Remove from the oven, turn the skewers and cook for an additional 5 minutes. The high heat of the oven should give the kebabs a nice sear.

9. Serve with lemon wedges.

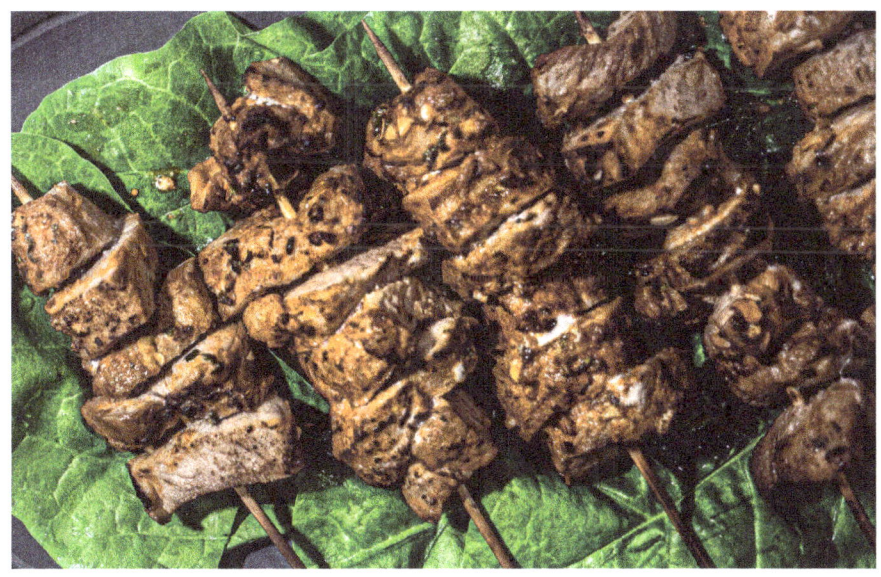

22. SIMPLE RACK OF LAMB

Cal.: 224 | Fat: 12g | Protein: 23.1g

Preparation Time: 60 minutes
Cooking Time: 4 hours
Servings: 2

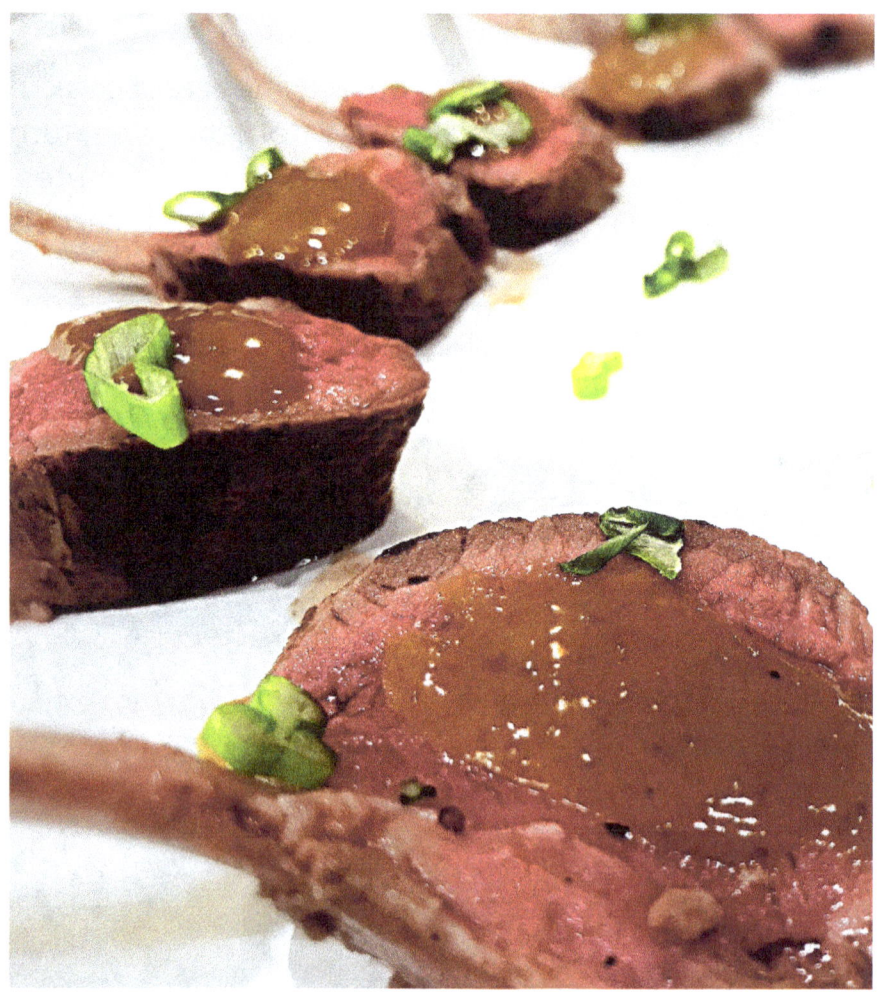

Ingredients

2 racks of lamb, trimmed
1 garlic clove, minced
2 teaspoons salt
1/3 cup fresh rosemary leaves
½ teaspoon freshly ground black pepper
2 teaspoons extra-virgin olive oil

Directions

1. Set your Sous Vide Machine to 134°F/56.5°C.

2. Combine the garlic, salt, rosemary leaves and pepper, and rub all over the racks.

3. Place the racks into separate vacuum-sealed bags. Marinate the bags in the refrigerator for 1 hour before submerging in the water bath.

4. Cook the racks in the water bath for between 2 to 4 hours.

5. When the lamb is almost done, heat your oven to 450°F/230°C.

6. Remove the racks from the vacuum-sealed bags and place on a baking sheet or roasting pan.

7. Roast in the oven for about 10 minutes. Remove from the oven and serve immediately.

23. BLACKENED BRUSSELS SPROUTS WITH GARLIC AND BACON

Cal.: 105 | Fat: 6g | Protein: 9g

Preparation Time: 16 minutes
Cooking Time: 85 minutes
Servings: 8

Ingredients

2 lbs. Brussels sprouts
3 garlic cloves, chopped
3 strips bacon
Bacon fat, from cooking the bacon
Salt and pepper

Directions

1. Preheat the Sous Vide machine to 183°F/83.9°C.

2. Wash the Brussels sprouts and use paper towels to pat them dry.

3. Heat a skillet on medium heat for a few min. When it's hot, add in the bacon. Cook the bacon until crispy, flipping halfway through. Remove the bacon and add in the garlic

4. Cook the garlic in the pan with the bacon fat until fragrant, about 1 minute. Then place the bacon fat and garlic in a bowl.

5. Put the Brussels sprouts in the bag or bags you're going to use to sous, along with the bacon fat, a little fresh ground pepper and garlic. Shake the bag around so everything is well mixed and seal the bag.

6. Place the bag in your preheated water and set the timer for 50 minutes.

7. At the 35-minute mark preheat your oven to 400°F/205°C and line a large rimmed baking sheet with parchment paper.

8. Place the cooked mixture on the baking sheet, making sure the Brussels sprouts are in a single layer. Put the baking sheet in the oven and cook the Brussels sprouts for 5 to 7 min. The sprouts should blacken a little bit when they're ready.

9. Serve immediately.

24. HUEVOS RANCHEROS

Cal.: 554 | Fat: 34.6g | Protein: 28.5g

Preparation Time: 11 minutes
Cooking Time: 2 hours 30 minutes
Servings: 3

Ingredients

½ can (7 ounces) crushed tomatoes
½ small yellow onion, minced
2 garlic cloves, minced
¼ teaspoon dried oregano
¼ teaspoon ground cumin
½ lime juice
1 canned chipotle adobo chili, minced
½ can refried beans
6 eggs
6 corn tortillas
¼ cup fresh cilantro, chopped
½ cup crumbled vegan cotija cheese or grated vegan Monterey Jack

Directions

1. Preheat the water bath to 147°F/64°C.

2. Combine tomatoes, onion, garlic, oregano, cumin, lime and chili in a bag. Seal using the water method.

3. Pour refried beans into a second bag and seal using the water method. Place eggs in a third bag and seal using the water method.

4. Place all three bags into the water bath. Cook for 2 hours.

5. When the other components have 20 minutes left to cook, heat tortillas in a pan. Place 2 on each plate.

6. Top the tortillas with salsa, followed by the shelled eggs, cheese and cilantro. Serve with refried beans.

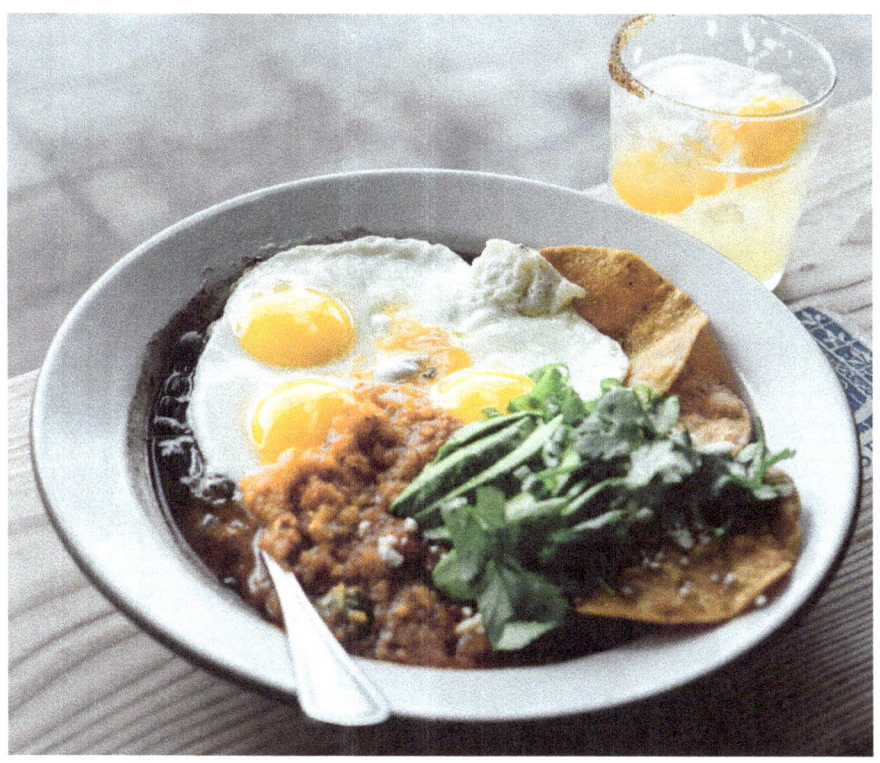

25. CHERRY TOMATOES WITH EGGS

Cal.: 210 | Fat: 6g | Protein: 12g

Preparation Time: 10 minutes
Cooking Time: 40 minutes
Servings: 4

Ingredients

1 cup cherry tomatoes, cubed
1 tablespoon ginger, grated
4 eggs, whisked
A drizzle of olive oil
1 red onion, chopped
Salt and black pepper to the taste
A pinch of red pepper, crushed
1 garlic clove, minced
1 tablespoon chives, chopped

Directions

1. Prepare your sous-vide water bath to a temperature of 170°F/76°C.

2. Pour oil in a pan and place it over medium to high heat.

3. Add the above-listed ingredients in the pan except

for the eggs.

4. Thoroughly stir the mixture and cook for 10 minutes.

5. Remove the pan from the heat and combine the ginger mixture with the eggs in a bowl.

6. Pour the mixture in a Ziploc bag and vacuum seal it after squeezing out the excess air.

7. Lower the bag into the water bath and cook for 30 minutes.

8. Once done, remove the bag from the water bath and serve.

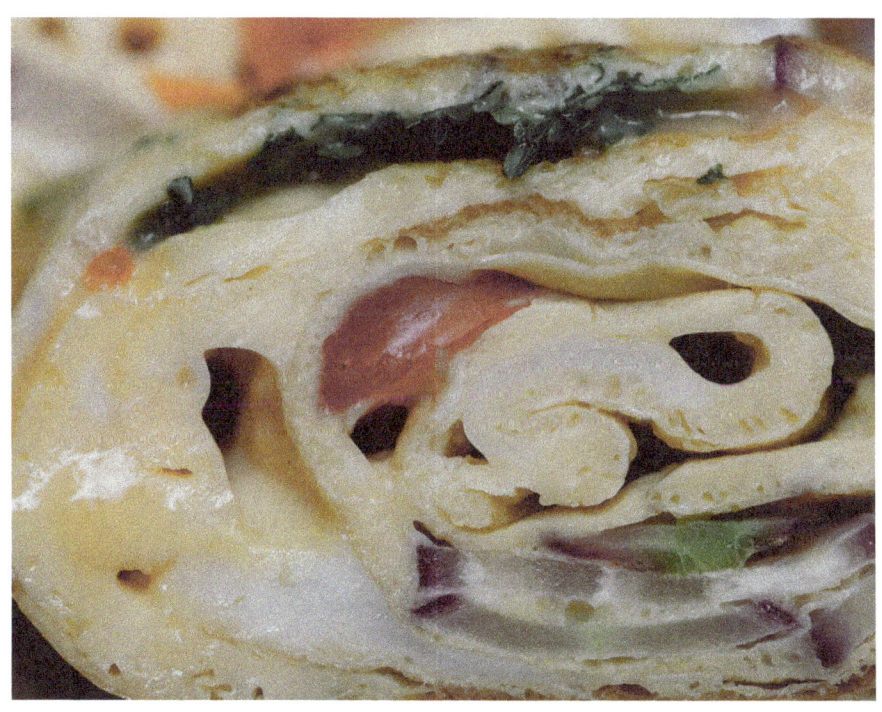

26. SHRIMP AND MUSHROOMS

Cal.: 340 | Fat: 23g | Protein: 17g

Preparation Time: 11 minutes
Cooking Time: 30 minutes
Servings: 4

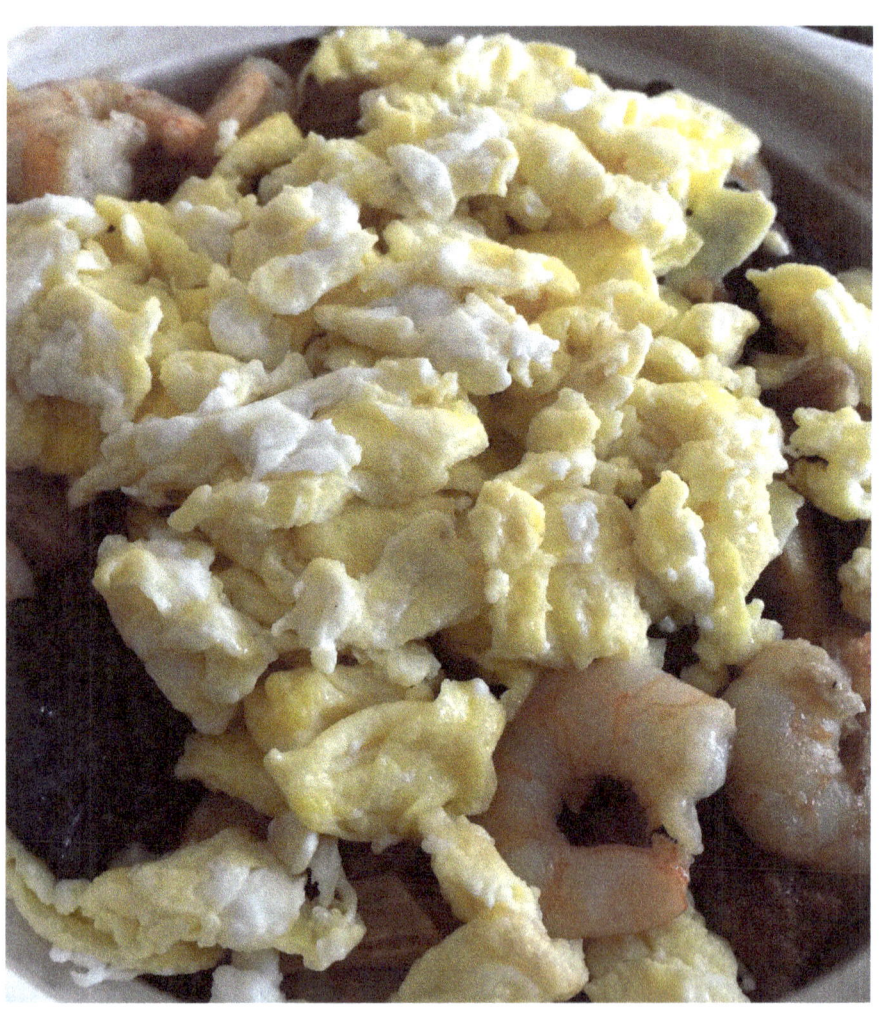

Ingredients

1 cup shrimp, peeled and deveined
3 spring onions, chopped
1 cup mushrooms, sliced
4 eggs, whisked
½ teaspoon coriander, ground
Salt and black pepper to the taste
½ cup coconut cream
½ teaspoon turmeric powder
4 bacon slices, chopped

Directions

1. Prepare your sous-vide water bath to a temperature of 140°F/60°C.

2. Vacuum seal all the listed ingredients and lower the pouch in the water bath.

3. Cook for 30 minutes.

4. Serve and enjoy!

27. SWEET PAPRIKA WITH ZUCCHINI PROSCIUTTO

Cal.: 200 | Fat: 3g | Protein: 10g

Preparation Time: 9 minutes
Cooking Time: 32 minutes
Servings: 4

Ingredients

1 teaspoon sweet paprika
½ teaspoon rosemary, dried
2 zucchinis, cubed
Salt and black pepper to the taste
4 prosciutto slices, chopped
8 eggs, whisked
¼ cup chives, chopped

Directions

1. Prepare your sous-vide water bath to a temperature of 170°F/76°C.

2. Put the eggs in a cooking pouch together with the other listed ingredients and shake to mix.

3. Vacuum seal the pouch and immerse it into the preheated water bath.

4. Cook for 30 minutes.

5. Remove the pouch from the water bath once cooked and transfer the contents to a platter.

6. Serve and enjoy!

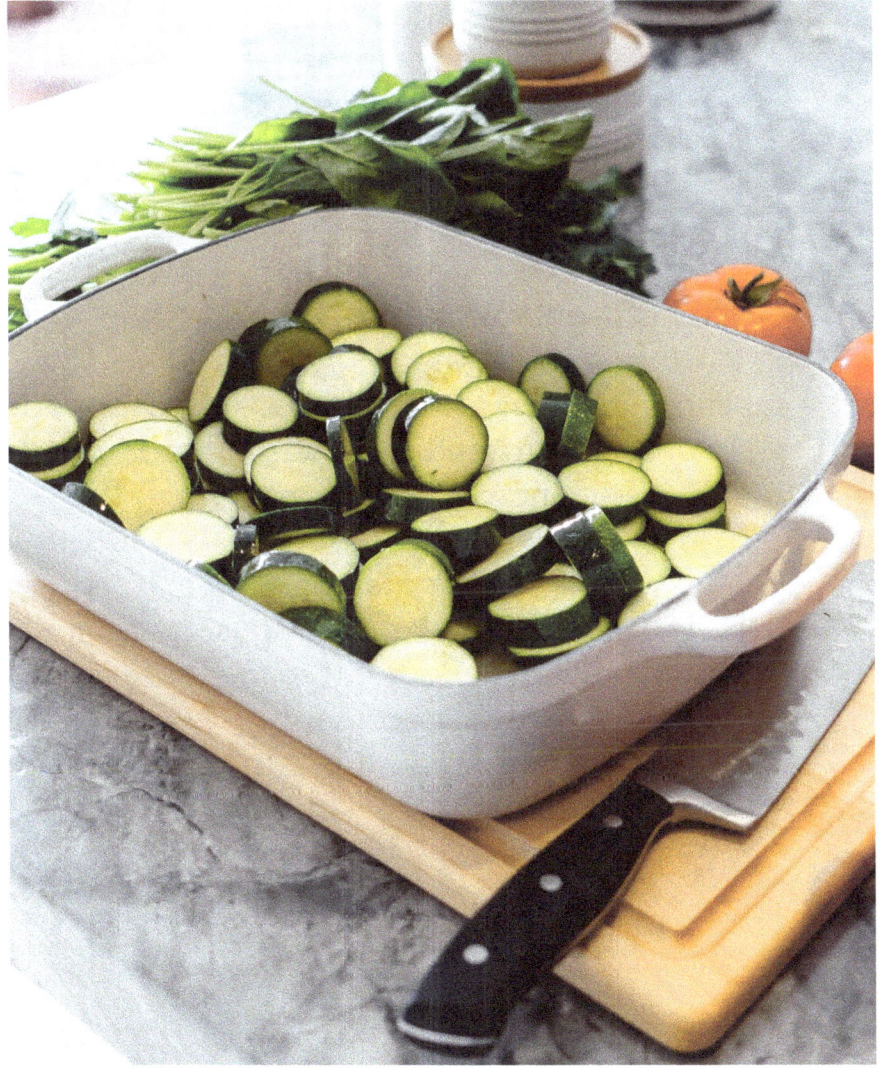

28. SPRING VEGETABLE RISOTTO

Cal.: 135 | Fat: 17g | Protein: 9g

Preparation Time: 11 minutes
Cooking Time: 50 minutes
Servings: 4

Ingredients

Risotto:
1 cup Arborio rice
3 cups vegetable or mushroom broth
½ tsp. vegan butter
2, 4 oz. cans mushroom stems and pieces, chopped
1 sprig fresh rosemary, leaves minced
Salt and pepper to taste

Spring Vegetables:
1 lb. spring vegetables like asparagus, broccoli, peppers, summer squash, cut into bite-sized pieces, peeled if necessary
Salt and pepper to taste
1 to 2 tbsp. vegan butter
Fresh or dried herbs of choice

Directions

1. Preheat the Sous Vide machine to 183°F/83°C.

2. Place the risotto ingredients in the bag you're going to use to sous and the spring vegetable ingredients in a separate bag and seal them.

3. Place the bags in your preheated water and set the timer for 45 min.

4. Place the cooked risotto in 4 bowls and fluff it with a fork.

5. Mix in the vegan cheese and vegetables, and serve.

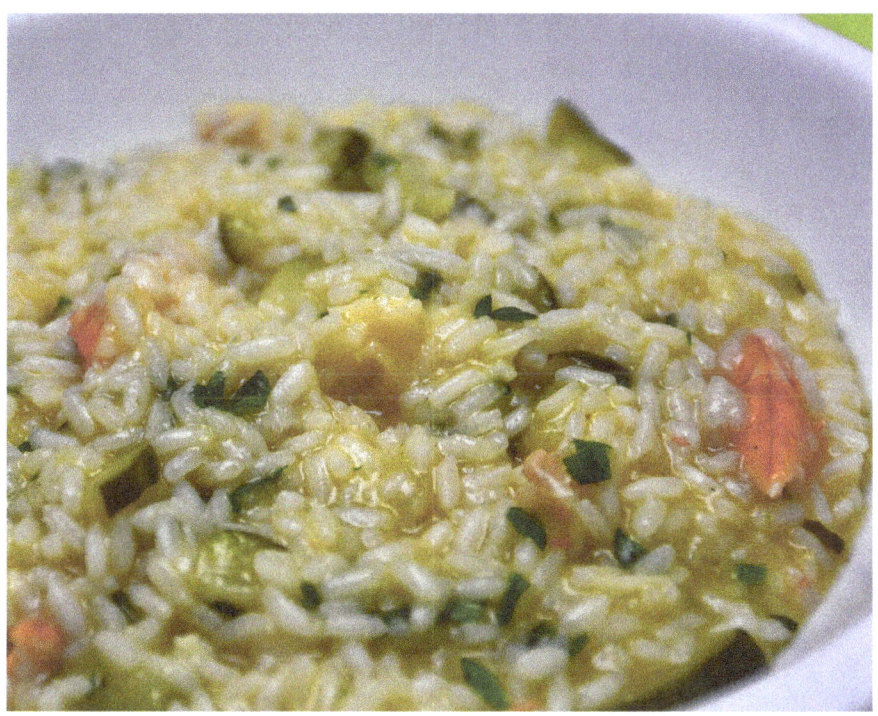

29. GARLICKY BRUSSELS SPROUTS

Cal.: 326 | Fat: 26g | Protein: 8.3g

Preparation Time: 21 minutes
Cooking Time: 1 hour
Servings: 2

Ingredients

1 lb. Brussels sprouts, trimmed
1/4 cup premium olive oil
2 tablespoons garlic, minced
1 tablespoon sea salt

Directions

1. Preheat a water bath to 185°F/85°C.

2. Add all ingredients to a bag and seal airtight.

3. Add to the water bath and cook for 1 hour.

4. Serve immediately with your favorite dish.

30. GREEN BEANS ALMONDINE

Cal.: 209 | Fat: 17.5g | Protein: 5.5g

Preparation Time: 15 minutes
Cooking Time: 90 minutes
Servings: 4

Ingredients

3 cups fresh green beans
2 tablespoons olive oil
1 tablespoon lemon zest
1 teaspoon salt
2 tablespoons lemon juice
½ cup toasted almonds

Directions

1. Preheat your water bath to 180°F/82°C. Clean and trim the green beans and mix with lemon zest and olive oil. Roughly chop the almonds.

2. Place the whole mixture in the bag, seal, and place in your preheated container. Set the timer for 1-½ hours. Put the cooked green beans on a plate, top with lemon juice, and season with salt.

3. Mix in the almonds and serve.

31. WINTER VEGETABLES

Cal.: 384 | Fat: 28g | Protein: 14g

Preparation Time: 12 minutes
Cooking Time: 58 minutes
Servings: 4

Ingredients

2 carrots
½ garlic clove
10 Brussels sprouts
1 small celery
2 salsify
2 parsnips
Rosemary and thyme leaves
Rapeseed oil
Rock salt

Directions

1. Peel the celery, parsnips, black salsify, and carrots and clean the Brussels sprouts. Depending on the firmness of the vegetables, cut them into more or less small pieces, halve the Brussels sprouts so that everything can be cooked at about the same time. Cut the garlic into fine slices.

2. In a large bowl, add the garlic and vegetables and

add the spices, oil, salt and herbs. Mix everything together well.

3. Put the seasoned vegetables in a bag and vacuum seal.

4. Preheat the water bath to 185°F/85°C and cook the vegetables for 50 minutes. Quench with ice water at the end.

5. The vegetables can now be kept for 7 days as long as they are in the bag.

6. If it is to be consumed, it is briefly swiveled in a wok or pan.

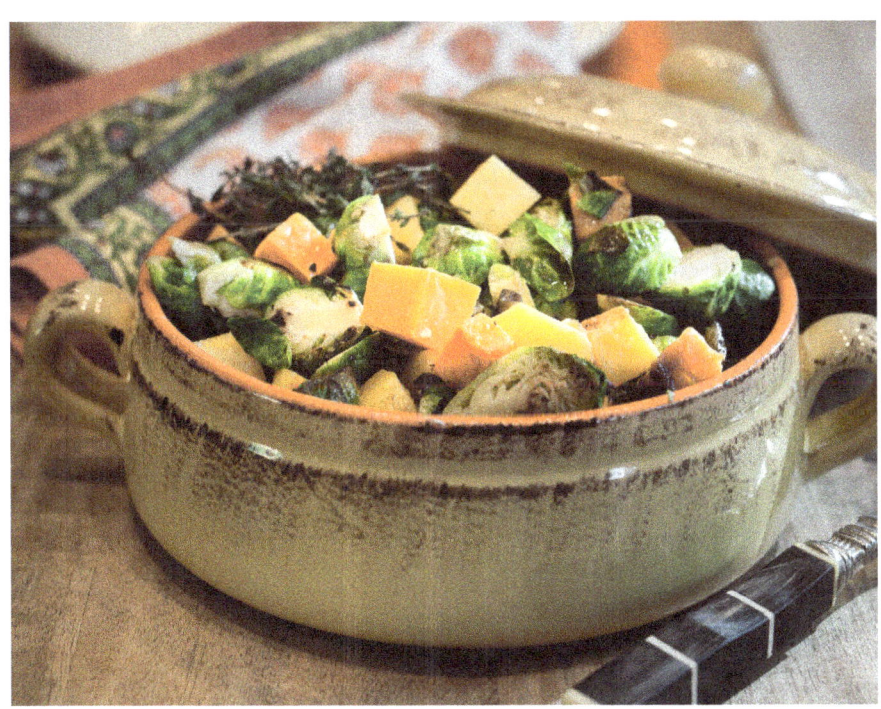

32. GARLICKY RATATOUILLE

Cal.: 264 | Fat: 18.6g | Protein: 5.3g

Preparation Time: 15 minutes
Cooking Time: 2 hours
Servings: 4

Ingredients

2 teaspoons red pepper flakes
1 yellow bell pepper, cored and sliced
1 eggplant, sliced
1 red bell pepper, cored and sliced
3 zucchinis, sliced
1 onion, peeled and sliced
½ cup tomato purée
Salt, to taste
10 garlic cloves, peeled and minced
5 tablespoons avocado oil
5 sprigs fresh basil, chopped

Directions

1. Prepare and preheat the water bath at 185°F/85°C.

2. Add veggies and all the ingredients to a zipper-lock bag.

3. Seal the zipper-lock bag using the water immersion

method.

4. Place the sealed bag in the bath and cook for 2 hours.

5. Once done, transfer the veggies along with the sauce to a plate.

6. Serve.

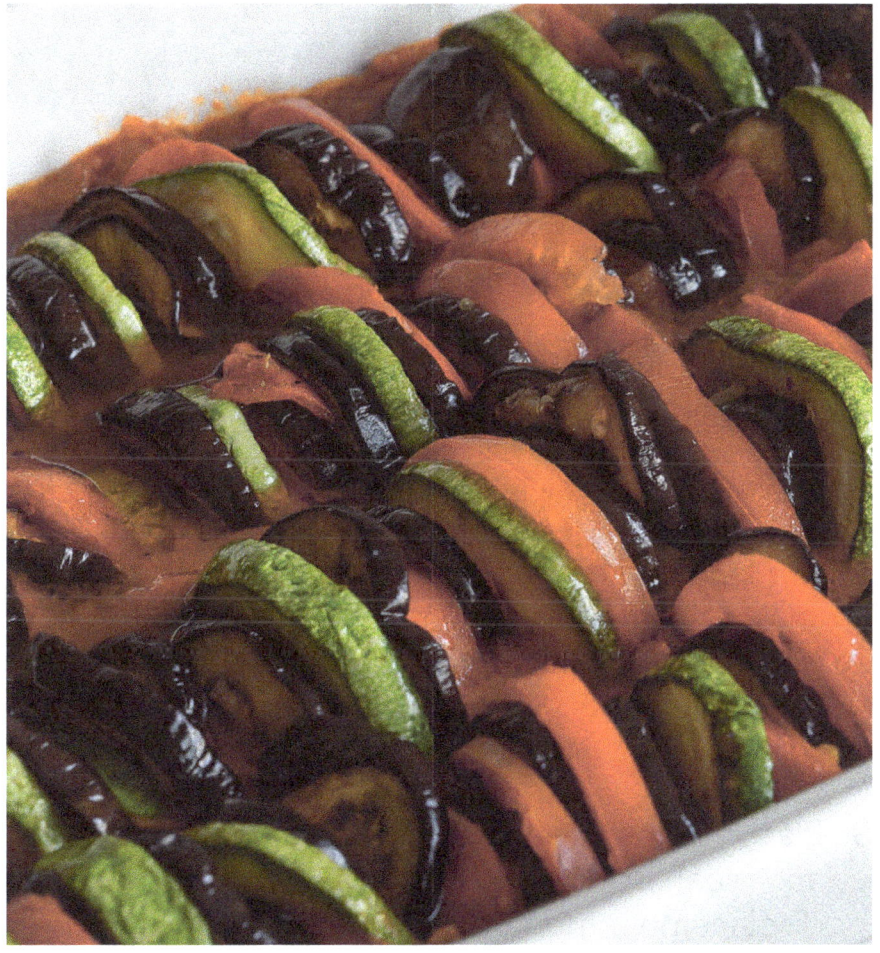

33. GARLIC MUSHROOMS WITH TRUFFLE OIL

Cal.: 332 | Fat: 34.1g | Protein: 1.5g

Preparation Time: 9 minutes
Cooking Time: 75 minutes
Servings: 2

Ingredients

10 media to large button mushrooms
2 garlic cloves, minced
3 tablespoons of olive oil
2 tablespoons of truffle oil
1 tablespoon fresh thyme, chopped

Directions

1. Prepare your water bath by attaching the immersion circulator and setting the temperature to 185°F/85°C.

2. Mix the olive oil with the truffle oil and the rest of the ingredients. Add the mushrooms and make sure that they are well coated with the oil mixture.

3. Place the mushrooms into a sealable plastic pouch and seal using a vacuum sealer or the water displacement method.

4. Place into the water bath and cook for 1 hour.

5. Once the mushrooms are cooked, remove from the bag, drain and toss in a grilling pan to sear, until golden brown.

6. Serve hot and garnish optionally with some extra thyme on top.

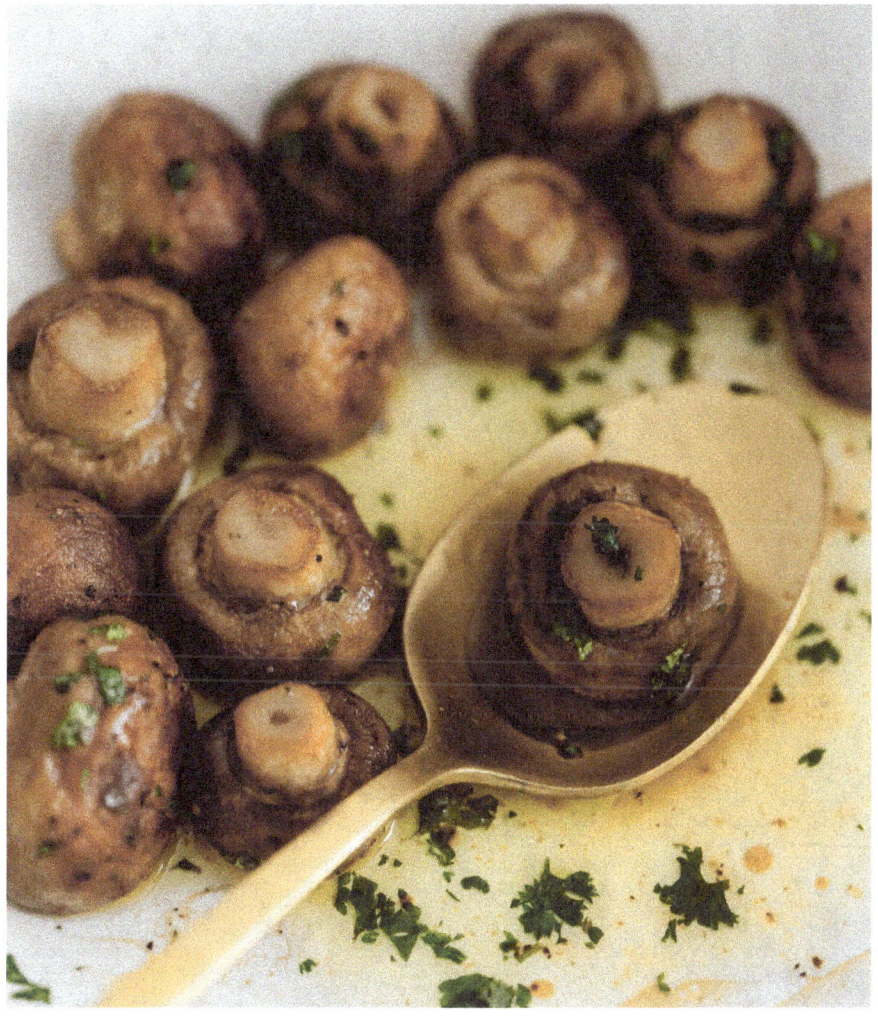

34. ROSEMARY POTATOES

Cal.: 269 | Fat: 26g | Protein: 14g

Preparation Time: 9 minutes
Cooking Time: 55 minutes
Servings: 2

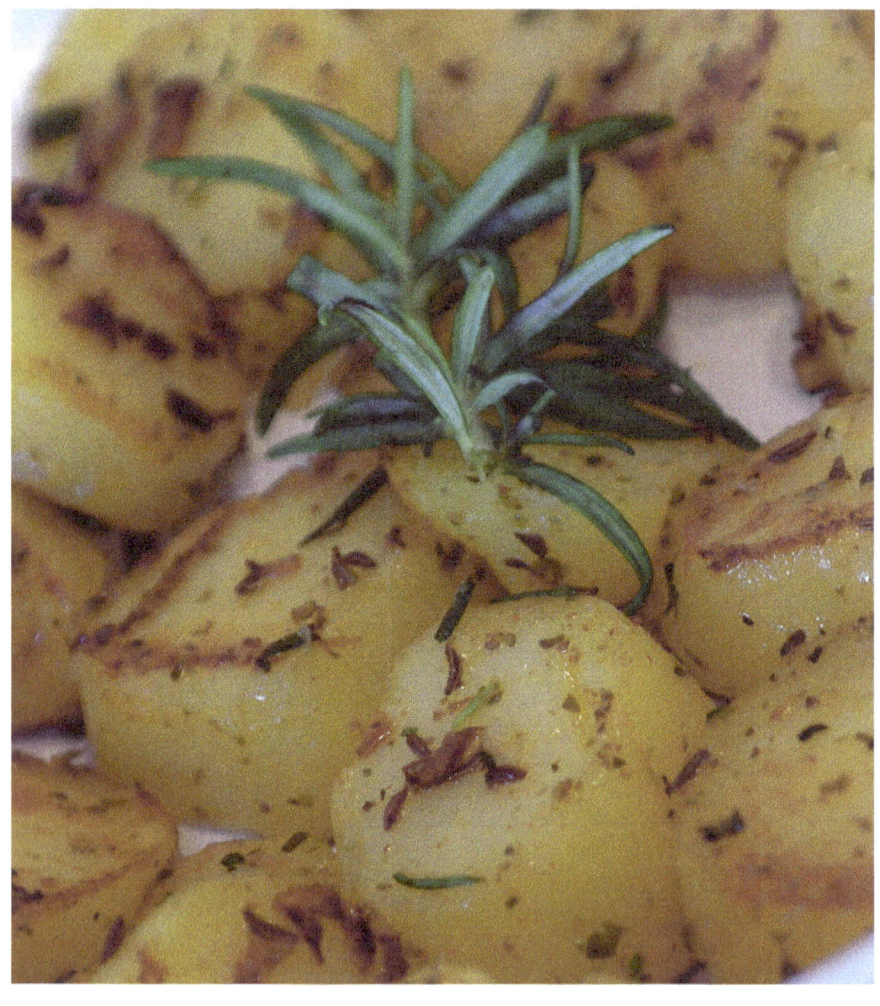

Ingredients

500 g potatoes
1 tbsp. olive oil
2 garlic cloves
1 bay leaf
1 sprig of rosemary
1 level teaspoon salt

Directions

1. Peel the potato and cut into smaller cubes.

2. Put the olive oil, salt, bay leaf, peeled garlic cloves and rosemary in a Sous-vide bag and seal it airtight with a vacuum.

3. Preheat the water bath to 185°F/85°C and cook the potatoes for 40 minutes. The cooking time also depends on the size of the potato cubes.

4. After the potatoes have been removed from the bag, they can be browned briefly in the pan until they are golden.

35. WARM ASSORTED BROCCOLI SALAD

Cal.: 93 | Fat: 3.4g | Protein: 5.6g

Preparation Time: 11 minutes
Cooking Time: 47 minutes
Servings: 4

Ingredients

3 heads broccoli, washed, chopped into florets
3 heads cauliflower, washed, chopped into florets
½ cup extra virgin olive oil, divided
20 cherry tomatoes, quartered
6 anchovy fillets, rinsed, cut into pieces
Salt to taste
Pepper powder to taste

Directions

1. Fill and preheat the water bath to 183°F/84°C according to the operating instructions.

2. Place the cauliflower and broccoli in a bowl. Sprinkle half the olive oil, salt and pepper. Toss well.

3. Transfer into a Ziploc bag and vacuum-seal it.

4. Immerse the bag in the water bath and cook for 45

minutes.

5. Meanwhile, place the tomatoes in a bowl. Add olives and anchovies and set aside.

6. When the vegetables are cooked, discard any liquid remaining in the pouch and transfer the vegetables into the bowl of anchovies.

7. Sprinkle the remaining olive oil. Add some salt and pepper. Toss well and serve.

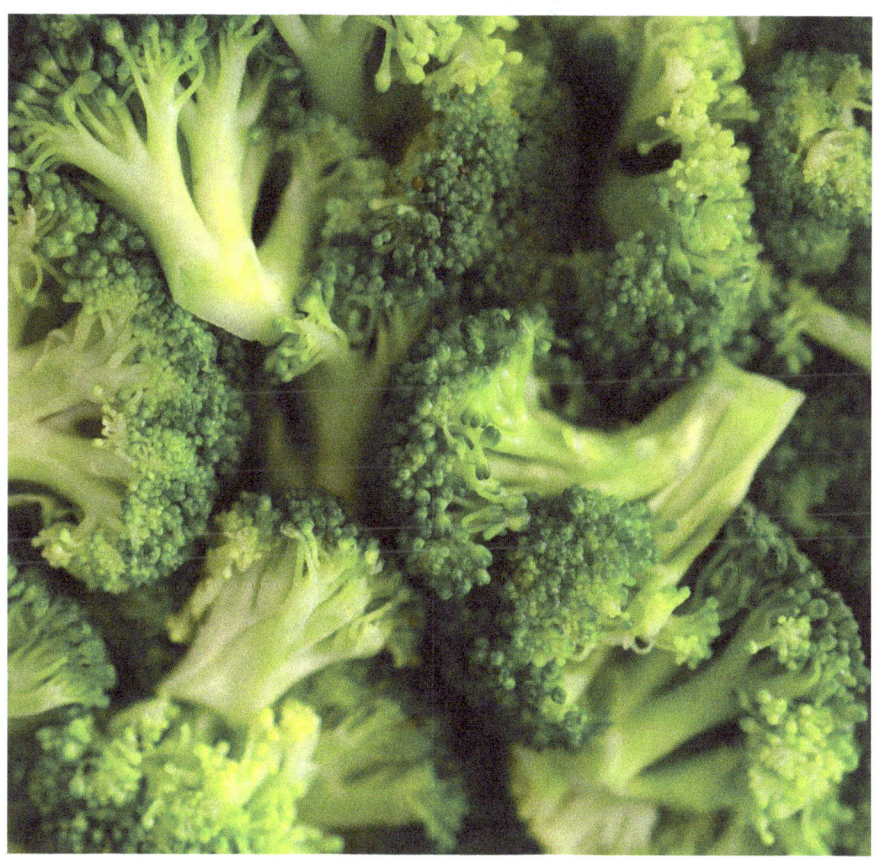

36. TANGY TENDER MUSHROOMS

Cal.: 90 | Fat: 7.3g | Protein: 4.1g

Preparation Time: 11 minutes
Cooking Time: 30 minutes
Servings: 4

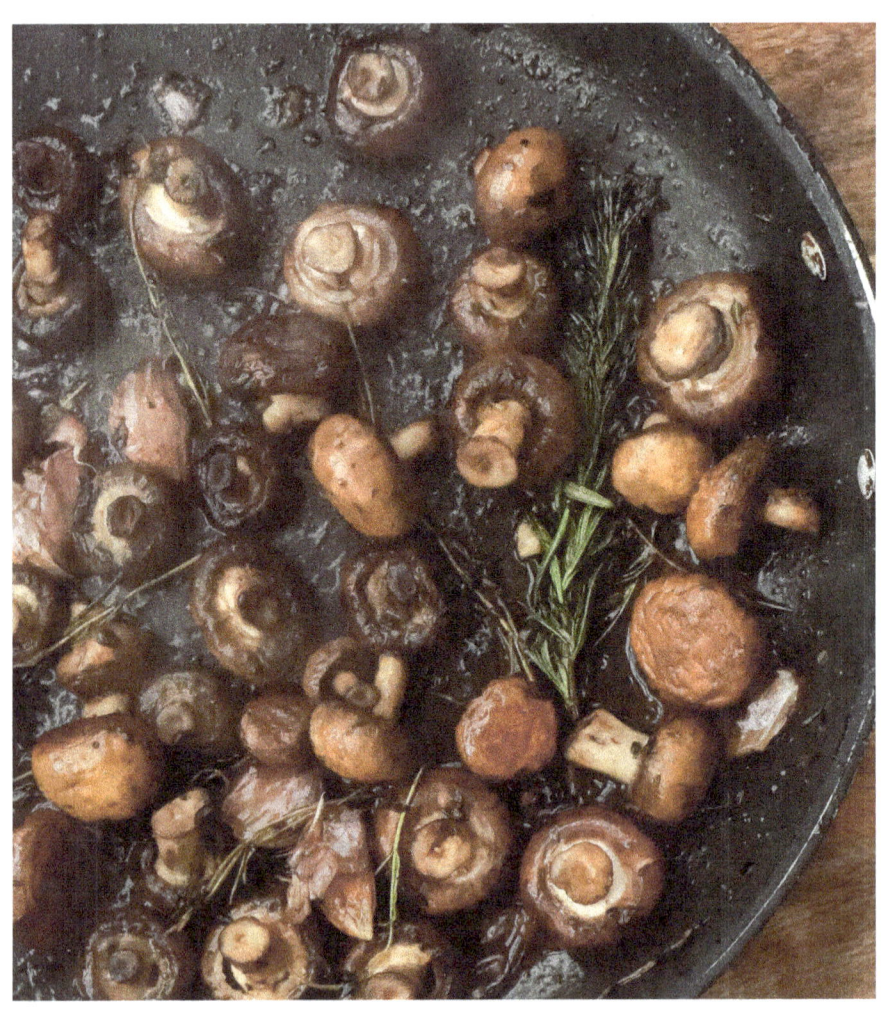

Ingredients

1 lb. button mushrooms cleaned, rinsed, and cut into bite-size pieces
2 tablespoons soy sauce
2 tablespoons extra-virgin olive oil
1 tablespoon balsamic vinegar
½ teaspoon black pepper
½ teaspoon sea salt, plus more to taste

Directions

1. Preheat your water bath to 176°F/80°C.

2. Combine the mushrooms with the rest of the ingredients, in a large mixing bowl, and toss to coat evenly.

3. Place the mixture in a sealable plastic bag; seal using the water displacement method or use a vacuum sealer.

4. Add mushrooms to the water bath and cook for 30 minutes.

5. Remove the bag from the water bath and serve immediately with your favorite meal.

37. COLORFUL BELL PEPPER MIX

Cal.: 31 | Fat: 0.4g | Protein: 1g

Preparation Time: 20 minutes
Cooking Time: 15 minutes
Servings: 2

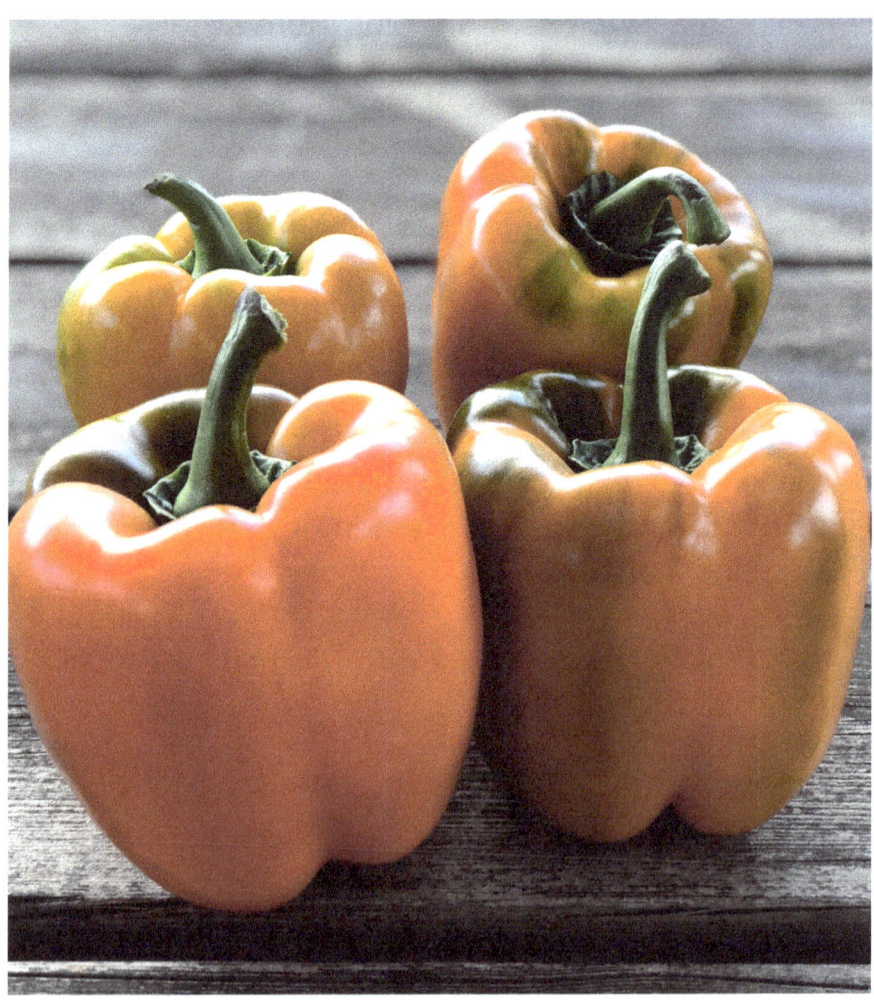

Ingredients

1 red bell pepper, chopped
1 yellow bell pepper, chopped
1 green bell pepper, chopped
1 large orange bell pepper, chopped
Salt to taste

Directions

1. Make a water bath, place a cooker in it, and set it at 183°F/84°C.

2. Place all the bell peppers with salt in a vacuum-sealable bag.

3. Release air by the water displacement method, seal and Immerse in the water bath.

4. Set the timer for 15 minutes.

5. Once the timer has stopped, remove and unseal the bag.

6. Serve bell peppers with its juices as a side dish.

38. KING PRAWNS WITH GINGER AND CARAMELIZED ONION

Cal.: 359 | Fat: 39g | Protein: 21g

Preparation Time: 14 minutes
Cooking Time: 30 minutes
Servings: 4

Ingredients

For King Prawns:
8 king prawns, skinned with their heads and tails
20 g ginger juice
For Caramelized Onions:
2 onions, thinly sliced
2 Tbsp. butter
2 Tbsp. balsamic vinegar
Pinch of sugar
Pinch of salt
1 Tbsp. thyme, finely sliced

Directions

1. Peel and cut the onions in half. Then cut each half into thin slices.

2. Add the butter, balsamic vinegar, sugar, salt and

thyme to a pot and put over high heat.

3. As soon as the butter and sugar melts, add the onions.

4. Stir to combine and sauté for 5 minutes.

5. When all the liquid has evaporated (about 5 minutes), lower the heat.

6. Continue to cook, stirring more often, until the onions turn golden brown (about 15-20 minutes).

7. Set aside to cool.

8. Preheat your water bath to 149°F/65°C.

9. Place the king prawns, caramelized onion and ginger juice into a Ziploc bag and seal using the water displacement method.

10. Cook for 6 min at 149°F/65°C.

11. When finished cooking, remove the bag from the water bath.

12. Open the bag and spread the caramelized onion out on a plate and stagger the king prawns on top, drizzling with the cooking juices.

39. CARAMEL SHRIMP CHILI

Cal.: 340 | Fat: 31g | Protein: 29g

Preparation Time: 15 minutes
Cooking Time: 30 minutes
Servings: 4

Ingredients

1 cup cooked rice noodles
1 pound cooked broccoli
1 chopped green onion
3 tablespoon sugar
1 tablespoon water
1 tablespoon oil
3 garlic cloves
1/4 teaspoon crushed red pepper
1 tablespoon fish sauce
1 pound shrimp
1/4 cup cilantro
Salt, pepper

Directions

1. In a bowl, toss broccoli, green onion and salt.

2. In a saucepan, cook water and sugar until it starts to caramelize. Add ginger, oil, pepper, fish sauce. Add cilantro and pepper.

3. Preheat the Sous Vide machine to 195°F/91°C.

4. Take the shrimps in a bag and seal it.

5. Place this bag in the water bath for 20 minutes.

6. In a serving bowl, add the noodles, shrimps and top with broccoli.

7. Add the shrimps with sauce and serve.

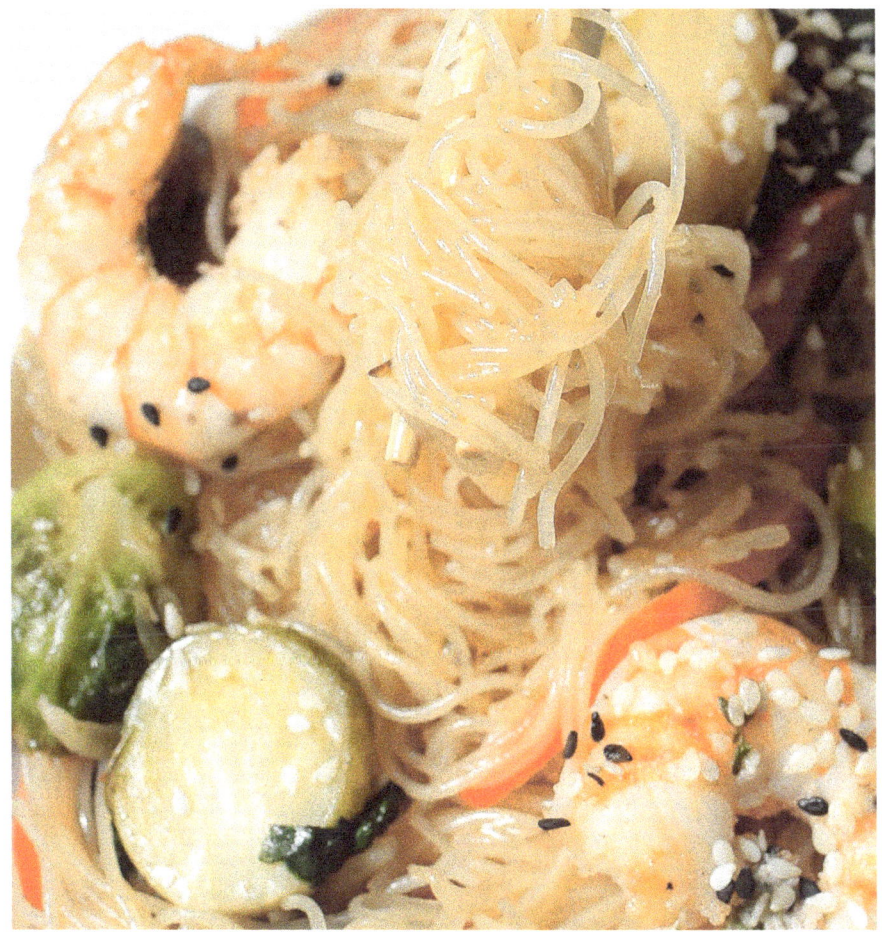

40. COD

Cal.: 329 | Fat: 38g | Protein: 16g

Preparation Time: 18 minutes
Cooking Time: 3 hours
Servings: 4

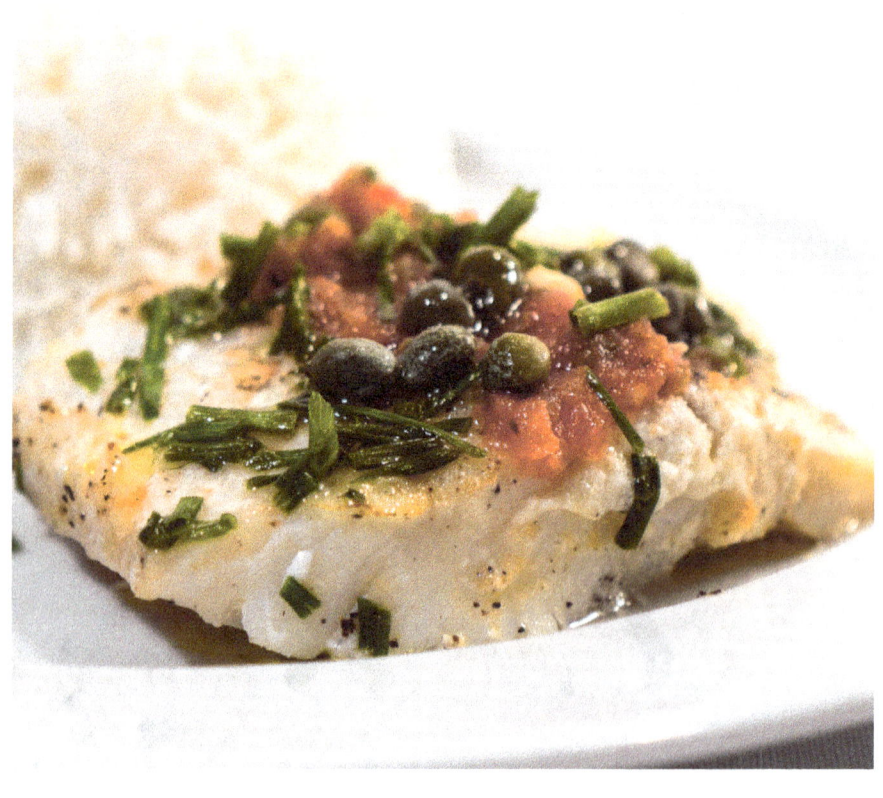

Ingredients

2 cod filets
2 Tbsp. vegan butter
1 sprig fresh dill
Lemon and Capers (Optional)
Salt, to taste
Pepper, to taste

Directions

1. Preheat the water bath to 131°F/55°C.

2. Place cod filets in a vacuum bag.

3. Add 2 tbsp. butter and sprig of fresh dill. Optionally you may also add a few slices of lemon and capers.

4. Seal the bag and cook for 30 minutes.

5. When finished cooking, remove from the bag.

6. Serve.

41. WALNUT COATED HALIBUT

Cal.: 359 | Fat: 39g | Protein: 21g

Preparation Time: 11 minutes
Cooking Time: 30 minutes
Servings: 4

Ingredients

2 Halibut Fillets
2 tbsp. Butter
Fresh dill, to taste
Lemon, to taste
Salt, to taste
Pepper, to taste
Olive oil, to taste

Directions

1. Generously salt both sides of the halibut and refrigerate for 30 minutes to 24 hours.

2. Preheat the water bath to 122°F/50°C.

3. Gently place the halibut fillets in a vacuum bag.

4. Add a bit of oil and fresh dill to the bag.

5. Seal the bag and place into the water bath.

6. Cook for 20/30 minutes depending on the thickness of the filet. We want to finish the Halibut in the pan.

7. Remove from the water bath and pat dry with paper towels.

8. Preheat a skillet pan with avocado oil on medium-high/high heat.

9. Add halibut, followed by a tablespoon or two of butter and fresh herbs.

10. Baste the halibut with butter as it cooks, 1–2minutes. You only need to sear one side.

11. Remove and serve!

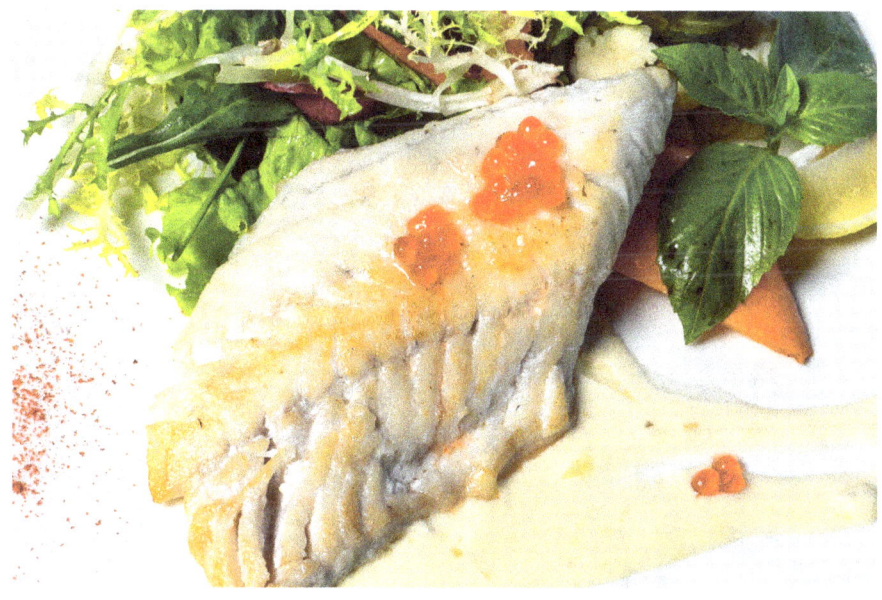

42. SALMON FILLETS

Cal.: 329 | Fat: 32g | Protein: 14g

Preparation Time: 12 minutes
Cooking Time: 43 minutes
Servings: 4

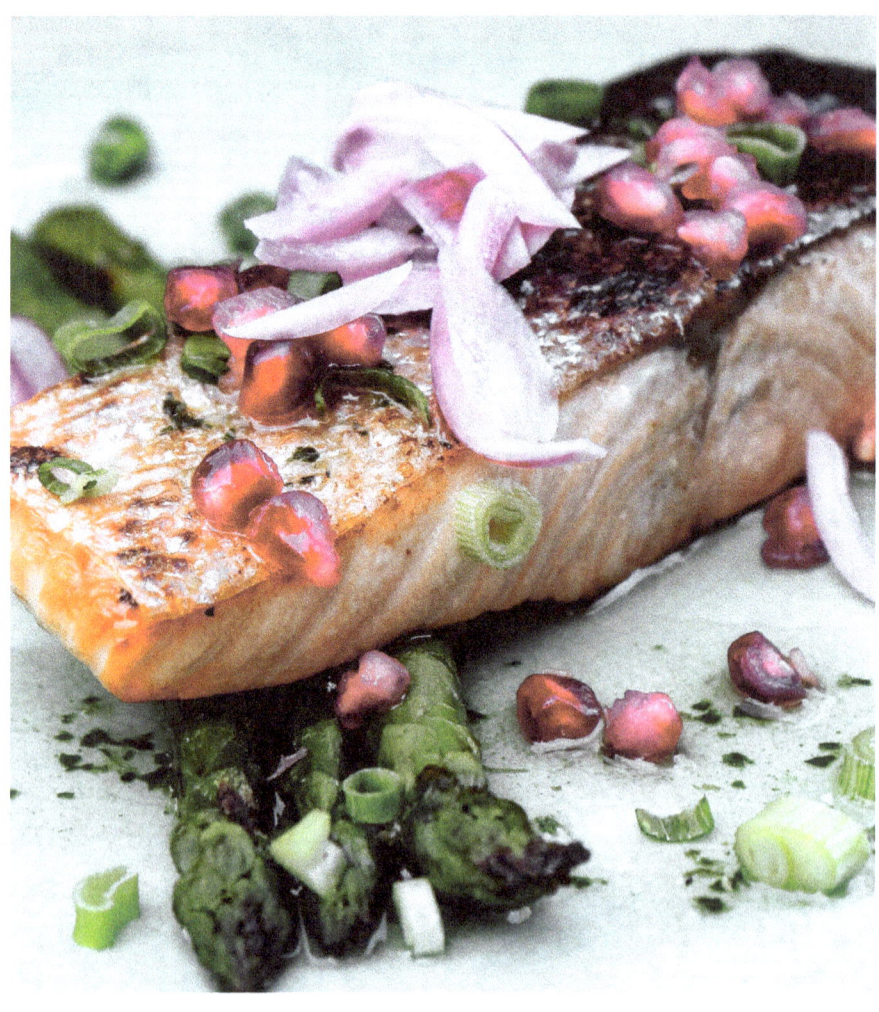

Ingredients

4 salmon fillets, each weighing approx. 130g
1 tsp. flaky sea salt
1 tsp. sugar
½ tsp. fennel seeds
½ tsp. coriander seeds
3 Tbsp. olive oil

Directions

1. Preheat the water bath to 122°F/50°C.

2. Lightly toast the seeds in a dry frying pan then transfer to a pestle and mortar. Roughly grind the seeds down a little

3. Place each salmon fillet in a vacuum bag with the seeds, salt, sugar and a dash of oil.

4. Seal bag and cook for 15 minutes.

5. Once ready, remove the fillets from the bags and drain on a paper towel.

6. Heat a non-stick pan with a dash of oil until hot then add the salmon skin-side down.

7. Cook until the skin is lightly golden.

8. Serve.

43. EAST ASIAN MARINATED CATFISH

Cal.: 463 | Fat: 38.3g | Protein: 23.7g

Preparation Time: 11 minutes
Cooking Time: 30 minutes
Servings: 4

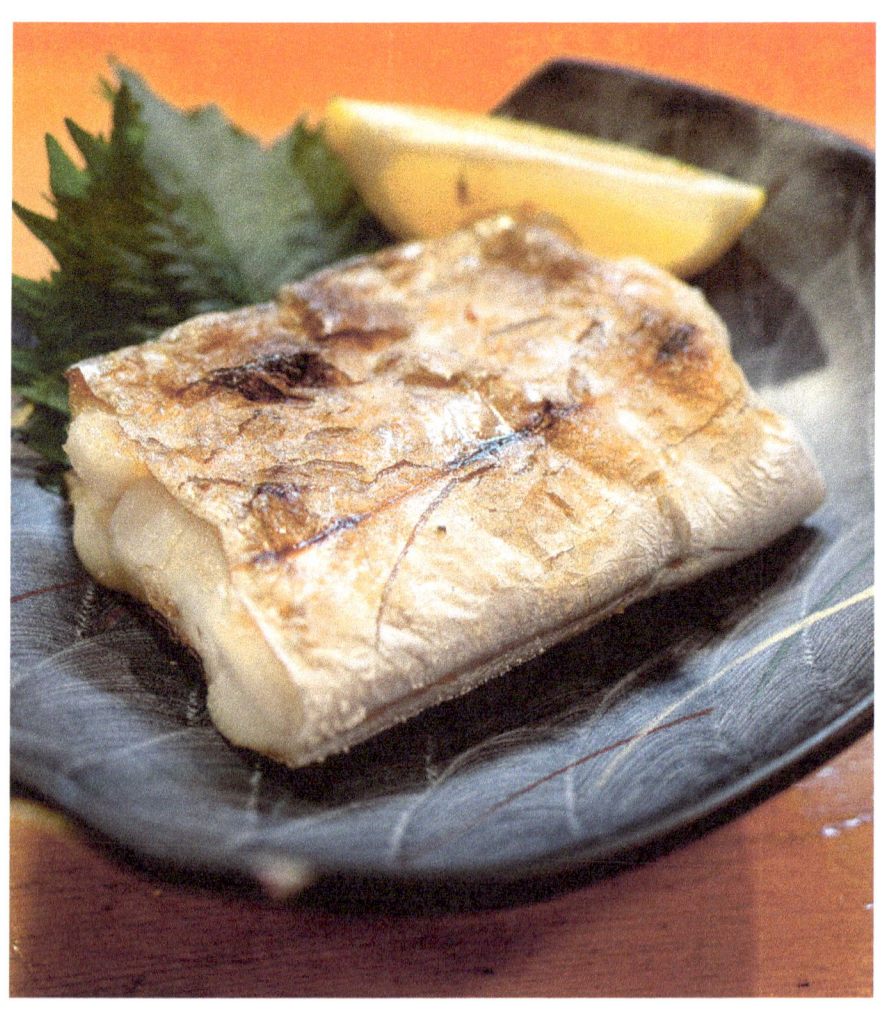

Ingredients

4 catfish filets
1/3 cup vegetable oil
1/4 cup low sodium soy sauce
2 garlic cloves minced
2 tbsp. rice wine vinegar
2 tbsp. sesame seeds
1 tablespoon sesame oil
1/4 tsp. black pepper
1/4 tsp. red pepper flakes

Directions

1. Preheat the Sous Vide machine to 150°F/66°C.

2. Combine all the ingredients in a bowl except for the catfish. Place the catfish in a bag, and pour the mixture in.

3. Place the bag in your preheated container and set your timer for 20 minutes.

4. When the catfish is cooked, serve it with the leftover sauce.

44. SIMPLE HONEY GLAZED CARROTS

Cal.: 145 | Fat: 24g | Protein: 16g

Preparation Time: 6 minutes
Cooking Time: 50 minutes
Servings: 3

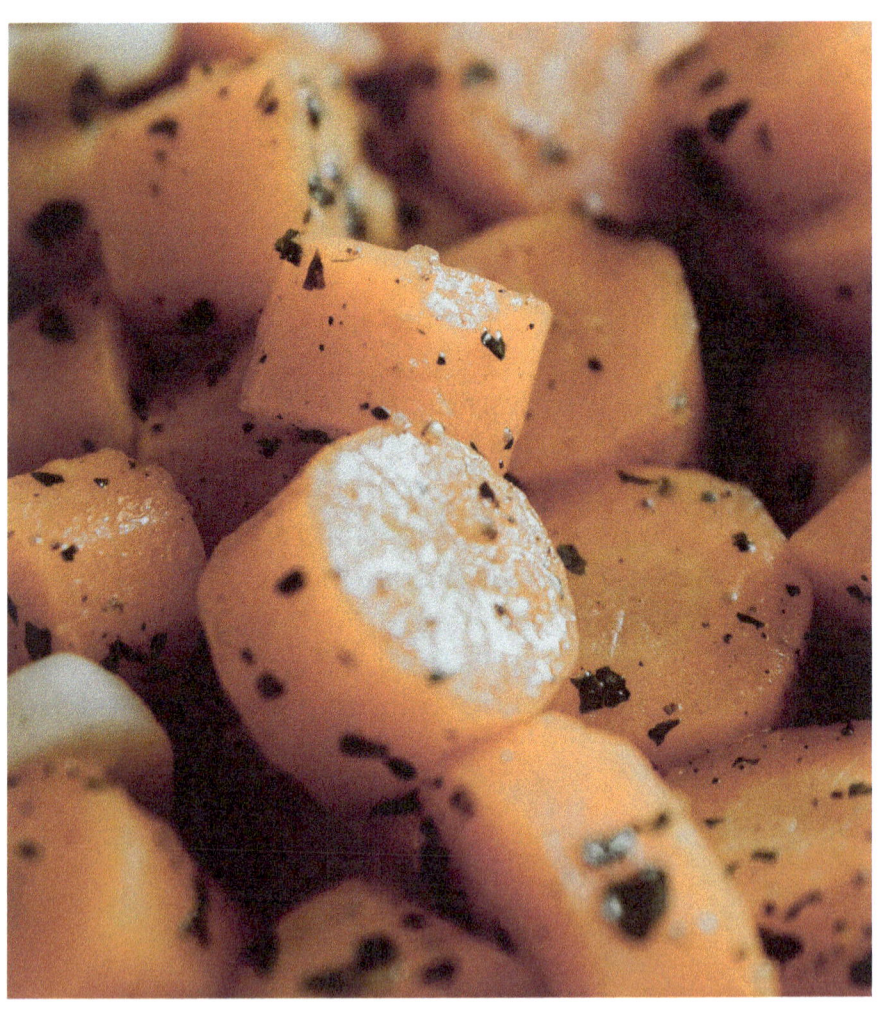

Ingredients

6-8 Medium to Large Sized Carrots, Washed and Peeled
3 tbs. Unsalted Butter
2 tbs. Honey
1 Cinnamon Stick
Sea Salt to Taste

Directions

1. Preheat the Sous Vide machine to 185°F or 85°C.

2. Place all the ingredients in the bag you're going to use to sous and seal the bag.

3. Place the bag in your preheated water and set the timer for 45 minutes.

4. Towards the end of the cooking process, heat a skillet on high heat until it's hot.

5. Place the cooked carrots in the skillet and sear for a total of 1 to 2 minutes, making sure to sear both sides

6. Top the carrots with a little more honey to serve.

45. SPICY PICKLED VEGETABLE MEDLEY

Cal.: 145 | Fat: 17g | Protein: 9g

Preparation Time: 11 minutes
Cooking Time: 30 minutes
Servings: 6

Ingredients

1 cup apple cider vinegar
½ cup sriracha
¼ cup granulated sugar
4 tsp. kosher salt
4 tsp. red pepper flake
1 cup baby beets, cut into quarters lengthwise
1 cup carrot, sliced ¼ inch
1 cup Persian cucumbers, sliced ¼ inch thick
1 cup shallot, sliced ¼ inch thick

Directions

1. Preheat the Sous Vide machine to 176°F/80°C.

2. Mix together everything but the vegetables in a measuring cup.

3. Place the beets in a bag, the carrots in a bag, and the cucumbers and shallots in a bag. Pour and an

equal amount of the liquid in each bag.

4. Place the beets bag in your preheated water. Set the timer for 30 min.

5. Add the carrots bag and cook the carrots bag for 15 minutes.

6. Add the cucumber and shallots bag and cook for 5 minutes

7. While the vegetables are cooking, prepare an ice bath, which is half ice half water.

8. Place the cooked vegetables, still in the bag in the ice bath and let it chill for 15 minutes before serving.

46. STRAWBERRY JAM

Cal.: 50 | Fat: 0.1g | Protein: 0.3g

Preparation Time: 11 minutes
Cooking Time: 90 minutes
Servings: 10

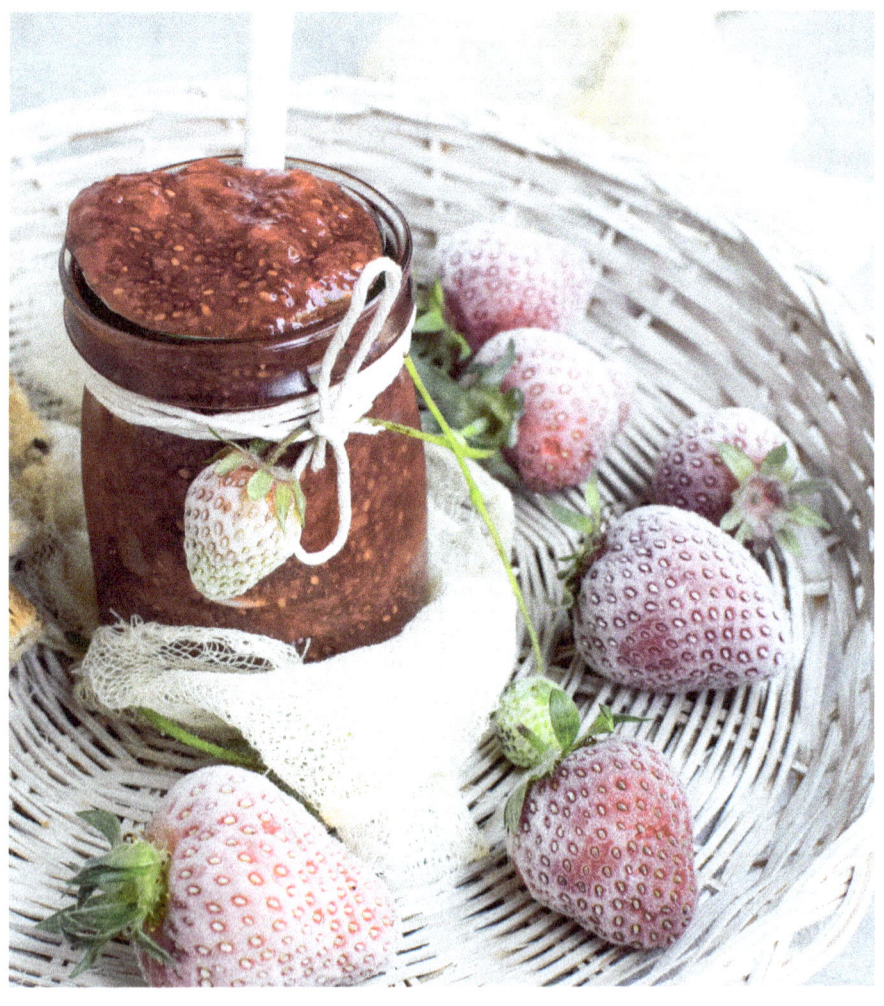

Ingredients

2 cups strawberries, coarsely chopped
1 cup white sugar
2 tbsp. orange juice

Directions

1. Preheat the Sous Vide machine to 180°F/82°C.

2. Put the ingredients into the vacuum bag and seal it.

3. Cook for 1 hour 30 min in the water bath.

4. Serve over vegan ice cream or vegan cheese cake, or store in the fridge in an airtight container.

47. STRAWBERRIES WITH BALSAMIC VINEGAR

Cal.: 72 | Fat: 0.4g | Protein: 1g

Preparation Time: 15 minutes
Cooking Time: 2 hours
Servings: 4

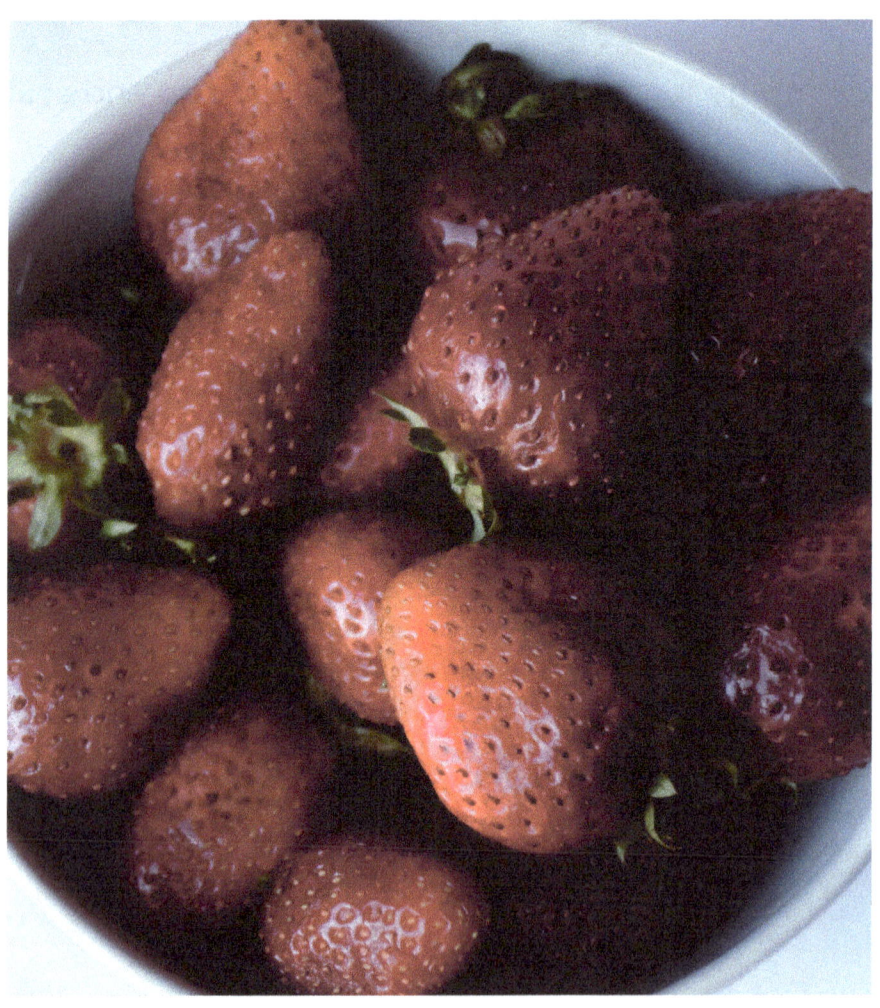

Ingredients

2 cups strawberries, quartered
2 tablespoons balsamic vinegar
1 tablespoon sugar

Directions

1. Prepare and preheat the water bath at 158°F/69°C.

2. Add strawberries and all the ingredients to a zipper-lock bag.

3. Seal the zipper-lock bag using the water immersion method.

4. Place the sealed bag in the bath and cook for 2 hours.

5. Once done, transfer the strawberries to a plate.

6. Serve.

48. ALLSPICE POACHED PEAR

Cal.: 245 | Fat: 1.1g | Protein: 1.1g

Preparation Time: 15 minutes
Cooking Time: 30 minutes
Servings: 2

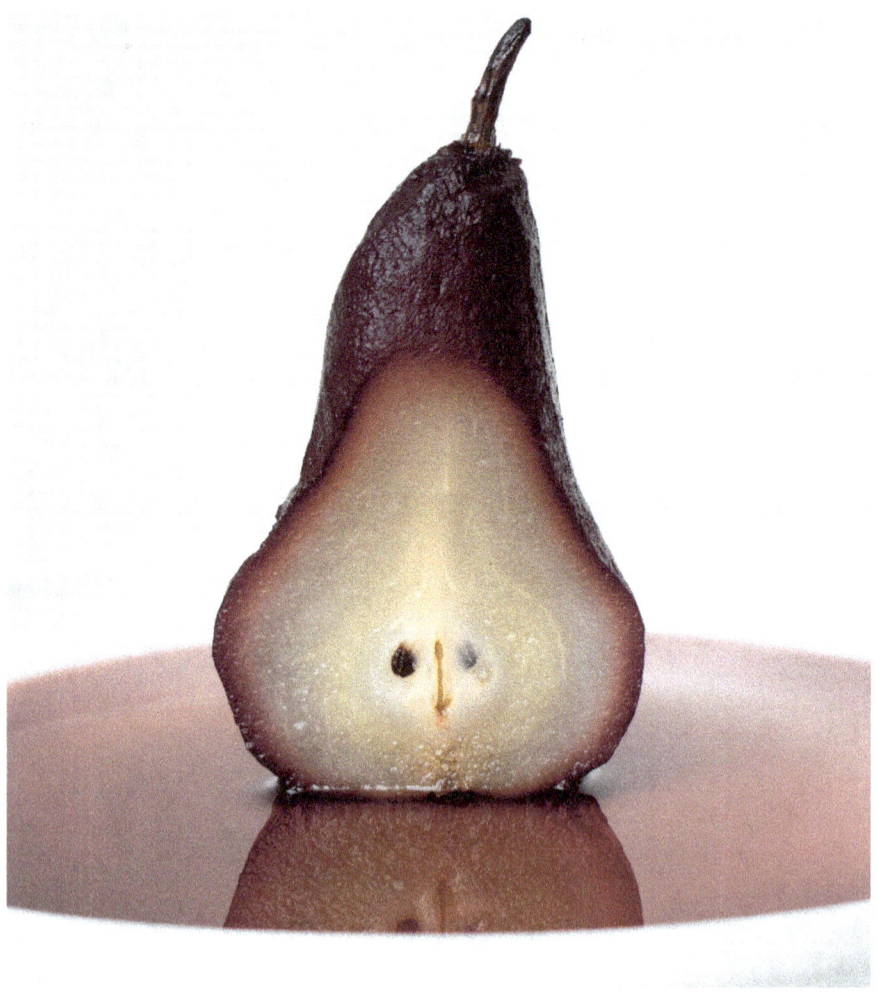

Ingredients

4 oz. red wine
10 oz. Sugar
3/4 oz. cinnamon stick, whole
1/4 oz. nutmeg, ground
1/6 oz. mace, whole
1/4 oz. clove
1/6 oz. allspice, whole
8 pears

Directions

1. Prepare and preheat the water bath at 176°F/80°C.

2. Add pears and all the ingredients to a zipper-lock bag.

3. Seal the zipper-lock bag using the water immersion method.

4. Place the sealed bag in the bath and cook for 30 minutes.

5. Once done, transfer the pears to a plate and slice them.

6. Strain the remaining sauce and pour over the pears.

7. Serve.

49. RASPBERRY COMPOTE

Cal.: 106 | Fat: 2g | Protein: 1g

Preparation Time: 11 minutes
Cooking Time: 60 minutes
Servings: 4

Ingredients

1 cups raspberries
1 lemon zest
1 orange zest
1 tbsp. white sugar

Directions

1. Preheat the Sous Vide machine to 185°F/85°C.

2. Put the ingredients into the vacuum bag and seal it.

3. Cook for 1 hour in the water bath.

4. Serve over vegan ice cream or cake.

50. CINNAMON APPLES

Cal.: 250 | Fat: 1g | Protein: 12g

Preparation Time: 11 minutes
Cooking Time: 70 minutes
Servings: 4

Ingredients

4 red apples, cored, peeled and sliced
4 tbsp. vegan butter
2 tsp. ground cinnamon
2 tsp. liquid honey
Juice of 1 lemon

Directions

1. Preheat the Sous Vide machine to 180°F/82°C.

2. Put the ingredients into the plastic bag, and seal it, removing the air.

3. Put the bag into the chamber and set the cooking time for 1 hour 10 minutes.

4. Serve warm in bowls with a spoon of vegan vanilla ice cream (optionally).

TEMPERATURE CHARTS

🥩 MEAT	°F🌡 TEMPERATURE	⏱ TIME
Beef Steak, rare	129 °F	1 hour 30 min.
Beef Steak, medium-rare	136 °F	1 hour 30min.
Beef Steak, well done	158 °F	1 hour 30min.
Beef Roast, rare	133 °F	7 hours
Beef Roast, medium-rare	140 °F	6 hours
Beef Roast, well done	158 °F	5 hours
Beef Tough Cuts, rare	136 °F	24 hours
Beef Tough Cuts, medium-rare	149 °F	16 hours
Beef Tough Cuts, well done	185 °F	8 hours
Lamb Tenderloin, Rib eye, T-bone, Cutlets	134 °F	4 hours
Lamb Roast, Leg	134 °F	10 hours
Lamb Flank Steak, Brisket	134 °F	12 hours
Pork Chop, rare	136 °F	1 hour
Pork Chop, medium-rare	144 °F	1 hour
Pork Chop, well done	158 °F	1 hour
Pork Roast, rare	136 °F	3 hours

🥩 MEAT	°F🌡 TEMPERATURE	⏱ TIME
Pork Roast, medium-rare	144 °F	3 hours
Pork Roast, well done	158 °F	3 hours
Pork Tough Cuts, rare	144 °F	16 hours
Pork Tough Cuts, medium-rare	154 °F	12 hours
Pork Tough Cuts, well done	154 °F	8 hours
Pork Tenderloin	134 °F	1 hour 30min
Pork Baby Back Ribs	165 °F	6 hours
Pork Cutlets	134 °F	5 hours
Pork Spare Ribs	160 °F	12 hours
Pork Belly (quick)	185 °F	5 hours
Pork Belly (slow)	167 °F	24 hours

🐟 FISH AND SEAFOOD	°F🌡 TEMPERATURE	⏱ TIME
Fish, tender	104 °F	40 min.
Fish, tender and flaky	122 °F	40 min.
Fish, well done	140 °F	40 min.
Salmon, Tuna, Trout, Mackerel, Halibut, Snapper, Sole	126 °F	30 min.
Lobster	140 °F	50 min.
Scallops	140 °F	50 min.
Shrimp	140 °F	35 min.

🍗 POULTRY	°F 🌡 TEMPERATURE	⏱ TIME
Chicken White Meat, super-supple	140 °F	2 hours
Chicken White Meat, tender and juicy	149 °F	1 hour
Chicken White Meat, well done	167 °F	1 hour
Chicken Breast, bone-in	146 °F	2 hours 30 min.
Chicken Breast, boneless	146 °F	1 hour
Turkey Breast, bone-in	146 °F	4 hours
Turkey Breast, boneless	146 °F	2 hours 30 min.
Duck Breast	134 °F	1 hour 30 min.
Chicken Dark Meat, tender	149 °F	1 hour 30 min.
Chicken Dark Meat, falling off the bone	167 °F	1 hour 30 min.
Chicken Leg or Thigh, bone-in	165 °F	4 hours
Chicken Thigh, boneless	165 °F	1 hour
Turkey Leg or Thigh	165 °F	2 hours
Duck Leg	165 °F	8 hours
Split Game Hen	150 °F	6 hours

🥕 VEGETABLES	🌡 TEMPERATURE	⏱ TIME
Vegetables, root (carrots, potato, parsnips, beets, celery root, turnips)	183 °F	3 hours
Vegetables, tender (asparagus, broccoli, cauliflower, fennel, onions, pumpkin, eggplant, green beans, corn)	183 °F	1 hour
Vegetables, greens (kale, spinach, collard greens, Swiss chard)	183 °F	3 min.

🍐 FRUITS	🌡 TEMPERATURE	⏱ TIME
Fruit, firm (apple, pear)	183 °F	45 min.
Fruit, for purée	185 °F	30 min.
Fruit, berries for topping desserts (blueberries, blackberries, raspberries, strawberries, cranberries)	154 °F	30 min.

WHAT TEMPERATURE SHOULD BE USED?

The rule of thumb is that the thicker the piece, the longer it should cook. Higher temperatures shorten the cooking time. Lower temperatures may take longer.

	TEMPERATURE	MIN COOKING TIME	MAX COOKING TIME
EGGS			
Soft Yolk	140°F (60°C)	1 hour	1 hour
Creamy Yolk	145°F (63°C)	¾ hour	1 hour
GREEN VEGETABLES			
Rare	183°F (84°C)	¼ hour	¾ hour
ROOTS			
Rare	183°F (84°C)	1 hour	3 hours
FRUITS			
Warm	154°F (68°C)	1¾ hour	2½ hour
Soft Fruits	185°F (85°C)	½ hour	1½ hour

	TEMPERATURE	MIN COOKING TIME	MAX COOKING TIME
CHICKEN			
Rare	140°F (60°C)	1 hour	3 hours
Medium	150°F (65°C)	1 hour	3 hours
Well Done	167°F (75°C)	1 hour	3 hours
BEEF STEAK			
Rare	130°F (54°C)	1½ hours	3 hours
Medium	140°F (60°C)	1½ hours	3 hours
Well Done	145°F (63°C)	1½ hours	3 hours
ROAST BEEF			
Rare	133°F (54°C)	7 hours	16 hours
Medium	140°F (60°C)	6 hours	14 hours
Well Done	158°F (70°C)	5 hours	11 hours
PORK CHOP BONE-IN			
Rare	136°F (58°C)	1 hour	4 hours
Medium	144°F (62°C)	1 hour	4 hours
Well Done	158°F (70°C)	1 hour	4 hours
PORK LOIN			
Rare	136°F (58°C)	3 hours	5½ hours
Medium	144°F (62°C)	3 hours	5 hours
Well Done	158°F (70°C)	3 hours	3½ hours
FISH			
Tender	104°F (40°C)	½ hour	½ hour
Medium	124°F (51°C)	½ hour	1 hour
Well Done	131°F (55°C)	½ hour	1½ hours

COOKING CONVERSION

TEMPERATURE CONVERSIONS	
CELSIUS	**FAHRENHEIT**
54.5°C	130°F
60.0°C	140°F
65.5°C	150°F
71.1°C	160°F
76.6°C	170°F
82.2°C	180°F
87.8°C	190°F
93.3°C	200°F
100°C	212°F

WEIGHT COVERSION	
½ oz.	15g
1 oz.	30g
2 oz.	60g
3 oz.	85g
4 oz.	110g
5 oz.	140g
6 oz.	170g
7 oz.	200g
8 oz.	225g
9 oz.	255g
10 oz.	280g
11 oz.	310g
12 oz.	340g
13 oz.	370g
14 oz.	400g
15 oz.	425g
1 lb.	450g

LIQUID VOLUME CONVERSION		
CUPS / TABLESPOONS	FL. OUNCES	MILLILITERS
1 cup	8 fl. Oz.	240 ml
¾ cup	6 fl. Oz.	180 ml
2/3 cup	5 fl. Oz.	150 ml
½ cup	4 fl. Oz.	120 ml
1/3 cup	2 ½ fl. Oz.	75 ml
¼ cup	2 fl. Oz.	60 ml
1/8 cup	1 fl. Oz.	30 ml
1 tablespoon	½ fl. Oz.	15 ml

TEASPOON (tsp.) / TABLESPOON (Tbsp.)	MILLILITERS
1 tsp.	5ml
2 tsp.	10ml
1 Tbsp.	15ml
2 Tbsp.	30ml
3 Tbsp.	45ml
4 Tbsp.	60ml
5 Tbsp.	75ml
6 Tbsp.	90ml
7 Tbsp.	105ml

LIQUID VOLUME MEASUREMENTS			
TABLE-SPOONS	TEASPOONS	FLUID OUNCES	CUPS
16	48	8 fl. Oz.	1
12	36	6 fl. Oz.	¾
8	24	4 fl. Oz.	½
5 ½	16	2 2/3 fl. Oz.	1/3
4	12	2 fl. Oz.	¼
1	3	0.5 fl. Oz.	1/16

RECIPE INDEX

Allspice Poached Pear 104
Arrowroot Country-Style Ribs 34
Bacon 48
BBQ Pork Ribs 42
Beef Tri-Tip with BBQ Sauce 36
Blackened Brussels Sprouts with Garlic and Bacon 56
Bourbon Chicken 30
Caramel Shrimp Chili 86
Cherry Tomatoes with Eggs 60
Chopped Duck with Honey 40
Cinnamon Apples 107
Cocktail Meatballs 16
Cod 88
Colorful Bell Pepper Mix 82
Crispy Egg Yolks 12
East Asian Marinated Catfish 94
Eggs and Oregano 14
Garlicky Brussels Sprouts 68
Garlicky Ratatouille 72
Garlic Mushrooms with Truffle Oil 74
Green Beans Almondine 69
Herb Rub Pork Chops 38
Huevos Rancheros 58
King Prawns with Ginger and Caramelized Onion 84

Lemon Herb Turkey Breast	32
Mushroom Orzo Green Soup	26
Potato and Curry Soup	28
Raspberry Compote	106
Rosemary Garlic Lamb Chops	46
Rosemary Potatoes	76
Salmon Fillets	92
Salty Custard	20
Shrimp and mushrooms	62
Simple Honey Glazed Carrots	96
Simple Rack of Lamb	54
Simple Sliced Pork Belly	44
Spiced Lamb Kebabs	52
Spicy Pickled Vegetable Medley	98
Spring Minestrone Soup	24
Spring Onion Soup	22
Spring Vegetable Risotto	66
Strawberries with Balsamic Vinegar	102
Strawberry Jam	100
Sweet Paprika with Zucchini Prosciutto	64
Tangy Tender Mushrooms	80
Tempting Teriyaki Chicken	50
Walnut Coated Halibut	90
Warm Assorted Broccoli Salad	78
White Bean and Artichoke Dip	18
Winter Vegetables	70

www.ingramcontent.com/pod-product-compliance
Lightning Source LLC
Chambersburg PA
CBHW070922080526
44589CB00013B/1404